A Flourishing Practice?

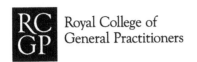
Royal College of
General Practitioners

A Flourishing Practice?

Peter D. Toon

The Royal College of General Practitioners was founded in 1952 with this object:

'To encourage, foster and maintain the highest possible standards in general practice and for that purpose to take or join with others in taking steps consistent with the charitable nature of that object which may assist towards the same.'

Among its responsibilities under its Royal Charter the College is entitled to:

'Diffuse information on all matters affecting general practice and issue such publications as may assist the object of the College.'

British Library Cataloguing-in-Publication Data

A catalogue record for this book is available from the British Library

© Royal College of General Practitioners, 2014

Published by the Royal College of General Practitioners, 2014

30 Euston Square, London NW1 2FB

Disclaimer

This publication is intended for the use of medical practitioners in the UK and not for patients. The authors, editors and publisher have taken care to ensure that the information contained in this book is correct to the best of their knowledge, at the time of publication. Whilst efforts have been made to ensure the accuracy of the information presented, particularly that related to the prescription of drugs, the authors, editors and publisher cannot accept liability for information that is subsequently shown to be wrong. Readers are advised to check that the information, especially that related to drug usage, complies with information contained in the *British National Formulary*, or equivalent, or manufacturers' datasheets, and that it complies with the latest legislation and standards of practice.

The views expressed in this book are those of the author and do not necessarily represent the views of the Royal College of General Practitioners, and should not be attributed as such.

Designed and typeset by wordtoprint.co.uk
Printed by Charlesworth
Indexed by Susan Leech
ISBN 978-0-85084-353-8

Where there is no vision, the people perish.

(Proverbs 2: 18)

Contents

Forewords

This book is the third in a series of texts that began with Peter Toon's Occasional Paper *What is Good General Practice?* back in 1994. Over two decades this series has documented Peter's sustained intellectual contribution to the discipline of general practice, refracting his front-line experience of both seeing patients and teaching young doctors through the lens of his fascination with philosophy in general and ethics in particular. The inspiration for his continuing meditation has been *After Virtue*, a book by the Scottish philosopher Alasdair MacIntyre that was first published in 1981 and which is now in its third edition. All those who, like me, have found wisdom and encouragement in Peter Toon's writing need perhaps to echo his own acknowledgement of Prof. Len Doyal, who first advised him to read MacIntyre. If only all such suggestions bore such abundant fruit.

The philosopher Richard Rorty described *After Virtue* as offering 'a diagnosis of the present state of moral philosophy which expands into a diagnosis of the present state of modern society'. Peter Toon's achievement has been to extend that diagnosis to the state of contemporary medical practice. He has expanded MacIntyre's description of the fragmentation of morality as a consequence of the Enlightenment and has created the marvellously rich metaphor of a shipwreck with all of us clinging to different fragments of moral theory that contradict each other, leaving us all in a state of increasing moral confusion. He then extends this metaphor to claim that 'people need sight of a lifeboat before they can abandon the philosophical flotsam to which they are clinging'. He offers a lifeboat kit founded on an ethics of virtue and applied to contemporary medical practice with an emphasis on the importance of internal goods for both patients and clinicians. Policy initiatives have been focused to a profoundly destructive extent on the external goods of money and power, and Peter Toon argues persuasively for a reassertion of the internal goods that constitute that sense of individual flourishing that is derived from the practice itself. He tests his arguments against the challenges of the Francis Report and offers us all as patients, clinicians and citizens a way of thinking and acting. He offers us a moral lifeboat.

Iona Heath

April 2014

In the 30-plus years since Alasdair MacIntyre first published *After Virtue* the reach of the book has been rather extraordinary, especially given its demanding analysis and its distinctly gloomy prognosis. Clearly our chaotic, fragmented culture still has a deep if inarticulate desire for Aristotle's *eudaemonia*, for a basic understanding of and increased capacity for human flourishing.

These ideas have a particular relevance for health care, partly because health, unlike many other good things, is a vital element of everyone's concept of a 'flourishing life'. And partly because of the alarming realisation that the NHS is losing its moral framework and drowning in an ill-amalgamated stew of incoherent and irreconcilable ethical fragments. This makes questions of what good health care might be, and how it might be delivered, important in themselves as well as offering a framework to look at how MacIntyre's 'virtue ethics' might be applied in practice.

Peter Toon does not argue here that flourishing requires a pain- and stress-free continuum from cradle to grave, an infinite extension of life and the abolition of inconvenience and effort. Rather he is suggesting that a 'flourishing practice' will deliver, to both doctors and patients, the enhanced capacity to perceive resilient and meaningful patterns in our lives, to develop virtues and to have a good death. (Here he does not take up in detail what might constitute a 'good' death; but I think he has set up terms with which to begin that discussion and I hope he, or someone else, will take it up soon.)

He focuses on which specific virtues (courage, compassion, justice, honesty, humility), both structural and personal, might best enable a medical professional, and particularly a GP, to develop these ends for her or himself, for colleagues and for patients. One of the things he sees as necessary is a stronger sense of collaboration and cooperation between doctors and their patients. So it is to his credit that as I read the book I found myself asking not 'Do I have a good doctor?' (I do) but rather, 'Am I a virtuous patient?' Do I come to encounters with my own medical practice with appropriate expectations, with proper hope, gratitude, humility, courage, willingness? What ought I to be bringing? How might I develop my capacity to be a part of this team?

These are questions I have never really asked myself before. I realise I have come to the activity of being 'treated' with a rather uneasy amalgam of self-pity and entitlement, given a slightly smug gloss by some infantile moralistic desire to be seen as someone who 'does not make a fuss'. As much as the doctor, I too need to learn to 'favour treatments that promote autonomy not as a right to be protected but as a capacity to be enhanced' and to contribute to 'our mutual and flourishing growth'. This feels demanding but meaningful.

Many years ago, Peter Toon was my, and my family's, GP. Through what turned out to be a very difficult decade for us all in many ways – with several medical difficulties – I know now we were consistently offered care that encouraged our flourishing. That is not why I am writing this foreword; that comes out of a subsequent history of other shared concerns and out of my desire to recommend this wise and helpful account. I mention it only because it gives an authenticity to my strong sense that Peter Toon 'speaks with authority and not as the scribes'.

I of course am a professional scribe, so do not take my word for it. Read this book.

Sara Maitland

April 2014

Acknowledgements

In the six years during which I have been intermittently working on this book countless people have said things or directed me to works that have been helpful, and unfortunately I cannot now remember all of these. I would however particularly like to thank Prof. Len Doyal for advising me to read *After Virtue* many years ago, and for Prof. Martyn Evans for writing his paper on the duties of a patient, because it was whilst reading this paper that the vision of *A Flourishing Practice?* came to me. I owe much to Prof. Gene Feder, not least for his encouragement to devote more of my time to ethics, without which encouragement I would not have given up my half-time academic post to have the time to write this book (the need for which is a sad reflection on the distortion of the practice of academic medicine). I am grateful to Jennifer Napier, Kim Stillman and John Spicer for comments on earlier drafts of this work, and to Helen Farrelly, Dr Rodger Charlton and the anonymous reviewers of the RCGP Publications Department, whose fresh eyes saw ways in which the nature and purpose of the work and some of the concepts used needed to be made clearer.

An earlier version of Chapter 3 was given at a conference on the Concept of Disease held at the University of the West of England in 2010, and much of Chapter 7 is based on the lecture I was invited to give at the RCGP Scotland conference on Compassion in Health Care in May 2013. During the writing process I also presented ideas from other parts of this work at several other conferences and workshops. I am grateful to the participants for their helpful criticisms and comments.

Very few of the ideas in this work are original; if it has any merit it lies in providing a framework that can bring the ideas of many other people together. I would like to thank all the many colleagues who have had the insights that I have attempted to collate, and who in a fragmented moral universe have nevertheless maintained the tradition of a flourishing practice.

Peter D. Toon

January 2014

Introduction

There is a constant stream of articles in the medical and the general press pointing out some moral problem or other with health care. Whilst preparing this paper I collected a thick file of these, a small proportion of which will be quoted in later chapters. I labelled the file half-seriously *'O tempora, O mores!'* Common themes within the genre include threats to continuity of care, inappropriate care at the end of life, problems associated with commercialisation and privatisation of health care, defensiveness and risk aversion, and unrealistic expectations of care.

The cry *'O tempora, O mores'* of course goes back more than 2000 years,[1] and is part of the human condition. As they get older every generation believes the country is going to the dogs. Are the articles in my file just the standard response of an older generation to things not being what they used to be, or do they reflect genuine problems in health care?

In fact by no means were all these articles written by older people, nor were they just written by doctors and other health professionals – a wide variety of lay people seemed to have similar feelings. And perhaps in the end to make the case that health care faces a moral crisis only one reference is necessary – the *Independent Inquiry into Care Provided by Mid Staffordshire NHS Foundation Trust: January 2005–March 2009*, the Francis Report.[2]

The view that health care is facing a moral crisis, in general or in specific ways, is often seen in terms of professionalism. A report on this subject from the Royal College of Physicians a few years ago[3] suggested that in society in general 'the ideals we equate with professionalism are in decline'. This report and other analyses of the state of medical care[4,5] suggest a number of factors that are contributing to this decline. Some are specific to medicine, such as changes in working practices leading to loss of continuity of care, diminution of personal responsibility, loss of medical team structure and leadership by example, and an NHS 'blame culture'. Factors affecting society more widely include rising consumerism, risk aversion and a decline in stability and continuity of relationships and the trust that this builds.

The influential virtue ethicist Alasdair MacIntyre however thinks that the problem lies deeper than this. In his influential book *After Virtue*[6] he suggested that our society has experienced a fundamental breakdown in the framework of our moral understanding, and that this is the underlying cause of the moral problems and uncertainties we face and which he argues affect all areas of our life, not just health care. MacIntyre believes that to resolve this problem our society needs a shared narrative, a shared tradition, and a shared world view. He suggests that shared social activities with traditions, which he calls 'practices', are a central support for these. One of MacIntyre's 'practices' is health care, or to be more precise medicine.[7] (I will consider the relationship between medicine and health care from MacIntyre's perspective in Chapter 2; for the present they can be seen as synonymous.)

The aim of this book is to try to see whether MacIntyre's analysis of our situation and his suggested solutions can in fact be applied to health care, and whether they might help resolve these problems in professionalism and the pervading sense of moral crisis.

MacIntyre, virtue and ethics

After Virtue is part of a renaissance of virtue ethics within philosophy in the late twentieth century. From classical Greece to the Renaissance, moral philosophy centred on the question 'What is the good life, and what do we need to do to live it?' Plato and Aristotle, but also the Stoics and Epicureans, devoted much of their attention to this question, as did the writers of late antiquity and medieval philosophy. For most of them the answer was phrased in terms of virtue – the personal qualities that we need to live well. Thomas Aquinas considered virtue to be a habit or disposition to act rightly. Although virtues are guided by reason, they are not merely a matter of the intellect – they involve emotions and motivation as well.

Moral philosophy conceived in these terms centres on *eudaemonia*. Flourishing is my preferred translation of this Greek word used by Aristotle and other philosophers when pondering the purpose of life. *Eudaemonia* is a key concept in virtue ethics, which is teleological – it argues that life has a purpose, it is a narrative with a meaning, and the purpose of moral philosophy is to work out the best shape of that narrative for each one of us. It is sometimes translated almost literally as the good life (the most literal translation is 'good spirited') and also as happiness. I prefer flourishing because it implies a life story that not only has a purpose but also a shape – periods of growth and development, full maturity but also decay and ultimately death. The word is commonly used of plants – flourishing like the green bay tree.

This teleological view contrasts with the view taken by consequentialism, one of the dominant ethical approaches in health care today, that life is a meaningless succession of good and bad experiences; and morality consists of trying to maximise the good and minimise the bad. *Eudaemonia* doesn't imply a life of uninterrupted fun, which would be neither realistic nor, probably in the long term, enjoyable – think of the soma-induced pleasures of Huxley's *Brave New World*.[8] A bland life of meaningless pleasure is not really a life worth living.

Aristotle and Aquinas, two of the greatest virtue ethicists, argued that we need virtues to achieve *eudaemonia*, to flourish. A virtue is a personal characteristic, a habit or disposition of the personality, a personal strength. Urmson[9] suggests that excellence is a better translation than virtue of the Greek word *arete* that Aristotle uses – not least because Aristotle discusses desirable intellectual as well as moral qualities. More recently Nussbaum and Sen[10] suggested that virtues are the qualities we need to overcome the challenges life throws at us.

But the virtues are also personal qualities worth having in themselves – the cultivation of the virtues is also part of the purpose of a good life. This is an important feature of virtue ethics, that being virtuous – having the habit of acting rightly, according to reason – not only enables us to do the right thing for others, but is also the best way for us to live too. It is a win-win approach; it's good news for everybody. This contrasts with rights and duties based on or not on deontological morality, the other ethical approach commonly used in health care, which is a zero-sum game – the more rights the patient has, the more burdensome duties the clinician has.

Virtue ethics is also more holistic than deontology or consequentialism. Unlike the Kantian dutiful person or consequentialist who considers the right thing to do according to duty or consequences then grits his teeth and does it, the virtuous person does what is right because it is in her nature to do so; she cannot do otherwise. Her emotions and indeed her whole being – body and mind – are directed towards doing what is right, so that it is 'second nature' and can be done almost unconsciously, just as an athlete's body and mind are trained and totally directed towards running a race. That of course doesn't mean the virtuous person doesn't think about right and wrong; *phronesis*, practical wisdom, is one of the cardinal virtues. But virtue ethics recognises that we are not just thinking machines, weighing up consequences or deciding what duty requires, but people with emotions that colour our experiences and motivate our actions; and that our bodies affect our feelings and thinking, too. In his comic novel *Three Men in a Boat* [11] Jerome K. Jerome remarked that a full stomach made him feel beneficent and at peace with the world; the Scottish Jesuit Gerry Hughes reported rather more seriously how tiredness and sore feet affected his response to people he met on his walk to Rome.[12]

Aristotle suggested that often a virtue lies between two opposite vices – the golden mean – thus for example courage is between cowardliness and foolhardiness.[13] Although in general this is a bit simplistic, we will find that this idea of moderation recurs throughout our discussion.

MacIntyre begins *After Virtue* with an account of the moral confusion we currently face and how it has arisen. In Chapter 1 I will look at some of the current problems facing health care (the things discussed in those 'O tempora, O mores' articles) to see whether they can be understood in the light of this account. This analysis suggests that MacIntyre's general critique of our moral framework does seem applicable to the problems health care currently faces.

In Chapter 2 I move on to attempt an account of health care as a MacIntyrean practice, particularly exploring the impact of this understanding of health care on the roles that patients and health professionals play in this practice. Here immediately we will find that MacIntyre's thesis leads to an approach to partnership between clinicians and patients no less real but somewhat different from that currently being promoted on a consumerist model. This discussion also involves thinking about the difference between an ethic with rights and duties at its heart and an ethic of virtue.

In Chapter 3 I will consider the internal goods of the practice of medicine. In part this will build on the consideration of the three aspects of general practice that I discussed in my first RCGP Occasional Paper.[14] It will also however involve consideration of the differences between a virtue ethic founded on developing a narrative of flourishing and a consequentialist ethic based on maximising the pleasure of a formless life. This has significant implications for the balance between the three elements of general practice. The interpretative function, often thought of as the 'extra' in medicine, in fact should be the centre of our practice. With this in mind, in Chapter 4 I will consider the boundaries of illness in relation to specific conditions. This reveals more ways in which health care is affected by a fragmented and confused moral discourse, and suggests some ways in which seeing the purpose of health care as developing a narrative of flourishing for individual patients may affect diagnosis and treatment.

In Chapter 5 I will explore the concept of professionalism and professional flourishing, and how this links to MacIntyrean concepts of internal goods and virtues. Chapter 6 deals with some of these virtues, particularly compassion, one of the key virtues that the professional in the practice of health care requires, and explores how they might contribute to flourishing. This understanding of professionalism is one of the key elements in considering the implications of a MacIntyrean position for the institutions that support the practice of medicine, including physical institutions providing health care, educational structures, continuing education and revalidation, which will be discussed in Chapter 7. Chapter 8 concludes the work with some brief suggestions on how we might start to move nearer to a vision of health care as a flourishing practice. This is more of an agenda than a prescription. This will include an analysis of the many limitations of the current work.

Few of the criticisms in this work of health care as it is currently practised or the visions of how things might be different are original; almost every week I find an article in the *British Medical Journal*, the *British Journal of General Practice* or the general media that makes one of the points found here. What I have tried to do in this work is to link these critiques and visions, fragments of the tradition of which MacIntyre speaks, within a coherent framework with a sound meta-ethical basis.

This is not a textbook of primary care ethics or a personal view of how health care should be organised; nor is it an evidence-based review of the current state of health care in the UK. Rather it is an attempt to use the philosophical approach of rational argument and the exploration of concepts and their implications to see whether MacIntyre's ideas might prove useful in addressing some of the problems facing health care today. It primarily deals with values rather than with facts, although these are so intertwined in health care that it is impossible not to take some view of what the facts are.

It takes important concepts one by one and explores them to see whether MacIntyre's perspective makes sense, and attempts to understand the implications of looking at the world of health care in that way. Also, like many philosophical works, it uses 'thought experiments' ('devices of the imagination used to investigate the nature of things'[15]) to try to imagine what health care would look like if MacIntyre's hypotheses were correct.

MacIntyre was pessimistic about the chances of piecing together a shared moral tradition from the fragments; he limits his claim for *After Virtue* to being a 'partial solution' to the problems we face.[16] Although this work too is at best a partial solution to the problems health care faces, I am less pessimistic than he is about the state of practices, certainly about the practice of health care. Much in health care in the UK today accords with his vision of a flourishing practice, although it is definitely threatened by the moral fragmentation he describes. Because it seems to me that a MacIntyrean approach can bring together many of the concerns commonly voiced about the way health care has been heading, it is worth giving some attention to how his ideas might work out in practice.

Notes

1. Cicero MT. *First Cataline Oration.* 63 BC. www.thelatinlibrary.com/cicero/cat1.shtml [accessed 16 January 2014].

2. Francis R. *Independent Inquiry into Care Provided by Mid Staffordshire NHS Foundation Trust: January 2005–March 2009. Volume 1.* London: The Stationery Office, 2013, http://webarchive.nationalarchives.gov.uk/20130107105354/http://www.dh.gov.uk/prod_consum_dh/groups/dh_digitalassets/@dh/@en/@ps/documents/digitalasset/dh_113447.pdf [accessed 16 January 2014].

3. Royal College of Physicians. *Doctors in Society: medical professionalism in a changing world.* Report of a working party. London: RCP, 2005, www.rcplondon.ac.uk/sites/default/files/documents/doctors_in_society_reportweb.pdf [accessed 16 January 2014].

4. Rosen R, Dewar S. *On Being a Doctor: redefining medical professionalism for better patient care.* London: King's Fund, 2004, www.kingsfund.org.uk/publications/on_being_a.html accessed [accessed 16 January 2014].

5. Levenson R, Dewar S, Shepherd S. *Understanding Doctors: harnessing professionalism.* London: King's Fund, 2008, www.kingsfund.org.uk/sites/files/kf/Understanding-Doctors-Harnessing-professionalism-Ros-Levenson-Steve-Dewar-Susan-Shepherd-Kings-Fund-May-2008_0.pdf [accessed 16 January 2014].

6. MacIntyre A. *After Virtue* (2nd edn). London: Duckworth, 1985.

7. MacIntyre. *After Virtue,* p. 194.

8. Huxley A. *Brave New World.* London: Chatto & Windus, 1950.

9. Urmson JO. *Aristotle's Ethics.* Oxford: Blackwell, 1988.

10. Nussbaum M, Sen A. *The Quality of Life.* Oxford: Clarendon, 1993.

11. Jerome JK. *Three Men in a Boat.* 1889. www.gutenberg.org/ebooks/308 [accessed 16 January 2014].

12. Hughes GW. *In Search of a Way.* Garden City, NY: Doubleday 1980.

13. Aristotle. *The Ethics of Aristotle: the Nicomachean ethics* (trans. JAK Thomson). Harmsworth: Penguin, 1955, Book II.

14. Toon PD. *What is Good General Practice?* (Occasional Paper 65). London: RCGP, 1994.

15. Brown JR, Fehige Y. Thought experiments. In EN Zalta (ed.), *The Stanford Encyclopedia of Philosophy* (fall 2011 edn). http://plato.stanford.edu/archives/fall2011/entries/thought-experiment [accessed 16 January 2014].

16. MacIntyre. *After Virtue,* p. 201.

Chapter 1

MacIntyre's fragmented moral universe and its impact on health care

Conceptual fragmentation

In the first chapter of *After Virtue*[1] Alasdair MacIntyre imagines an Orwellian future in which there is a Luddite reaction against natural science; laboratories are smashed and the culture of scientific discourse is destroyed. Some time later people try to recreate scientific knowledge, but all they possess are fragments, without any real understanding of the nature and purpose of science. So:

> *adults argue with each other about the respective merits of relativity theory, evolutionary theory and phlogiston theory, although they possess only a very partial knowledge of each. Children learn by heart the surviving portions of the periodic table and recite as incantations some of the theorems of Euclid.*[2]

He goes on to suggest that our understanding of morality and the language we use about it is in a similar state of disorder to that of science in his imaginary world. The destruction of tradition that he argues was a consequence of the Enlightenment has broken up the moral framework in which we live, as the wreck of a ship breaks up its hull. We are left with fragments, pieces of theory and their implications, which hold together in themselves but that are not connected to each other. We are clinging to this wreckage, but without the underlying consensus of a shared tradition there is nothing to hold the fragments together. This, he argues, is why many of our ethical discussions cannot be resolved; they are conducted between people clinging to separate bits of the moral wreckage, shouting at one another across a sea of chaos.

The debate on abortion illustrates this. Some believe that the fetus is a person just as much as any adult is. Like an adult it has a 'right to life', and any action that interferes with that right counts as murder.[3] Others argue that a woman has a 'right to choose'[4] whether or not to go on with a pregnancy she does not want and has tried hard to prevent.[5] Yet others believe that a decision on an unwanted pregnancy should depend on the likely outcomes of going on with the pregnancy or terminating it; sometimes abortion offers the best chance of happiness for the pregnant woman and/or her existing children, and so is best; at other times it does not. Each conclusion follows logically from its premises, but we lack a way to reconcile the differences between premises with conflicting outcomes; in philosophical jargon they are 'incommensurable'.

To test whether this idea is helpful in understanding the moral problems that health care faces we must examine the conceptual frameworks within which we currently organise our values. If MacIntyre is right then we will find separate 'fragments' of the moral shipwreck that do not fit together. This does seem to be the case. Much of the discussion of values in health care today can be seen as taking place within the framework of 'fragments' of moral discourse, each of which makes sense separately but which are not coherently related. An outline of one possible analysis of value 'fragments' and how they are used in health care, with some examples of how these seem to be used incommensurably to address some aspects of medical practice, forms the rest of this chapter.

The deontological fragment

Since the Enlightenment, approaches to ethics based on rights and duties (deontological) or on the results of actions (consequentialist) have dominated moral philosophy, and so it is not surprising that they are major influences in thinking about values in medical practice. Ethicists see the two as alternatives and there is much discussion of the rival merits of each, but health care appears to use them both, but for different purposes.

Deontological ethical systems are based on rights and reciprocal duties. Thus the right to life imposes on others a duty not to kill. This is a 'negative duty' (a duty not to do something) and it is linked to a 'liberty right'[6] – the freedom not to have harmful things done. There are also 'claim' rights, linked to 'positive duties'. Thus, for the right of children to education[7] to be meaningful, someone (parents, the local community or the state) must have a duty to provide that education; without someone with a positive duty to meet a claim, rights are just a rhetorical device, or as Bentham suggested 'nonsense on stilts'.[8]

The language of rights has become increasingly popular in recent years, particularly in the UK since the inclusion of the European Convention on Human Rights in our law by the Human Rights Act 1998.[9] The NHS constitution[10] is framed largely in terms of rights, most of which impose duties on health professionals or institutions that provide health care. Evans[11] suggested that health care might be more collaborative if there were more emphasis on patients' duties; interestingly, the NHS constitution uses the weaker term 'responsibilities' when discussing what is expected of patients. (This may reflect the influence of consumerism, another 'fragment' discussed below.)

Discussions of professional standards in health care are usually conducted in terms of duties. In the UK for medical practitioners the General Medical Council's (GMC) 'Duties of a doctor'[12] is central. Other professional codes are similarly phrased.[13] Although the Nursing and Midwifery Council Code[14] does not explicitly speak of duty, it mentions patient rights and uses a repeated 'you must' stem that is typical of deontological imperatives.

The language used in these statements has been criticised for lack of realism.[15] For some, duty is a gloomy word, the 'Stern daughter of the voice of God'[16] bringing to mind obligatory Sunday afternoon visits to boring aunts, sharing your chocolates with hated cousins and finishing your greens. We do our duty because we have to rather than because we want to. Indeed, some dour deontologists have suggested that an act only counts as good if you don't really want to do it. Visiting a friend in hospital because you care for him and enjoy his company isn't morally praiseworthy; it is acting according to duty but not from duty. This view is often attributed to Kant, although not all commentators accept this interpretation of his views.[17]

Certainly 'Duties of a doctor' can feel depressing. With so many demanding duties one may be excused for asking 'Why bother?' Someone with the natural gifts and educational achievements needed to practise medicine could surely have more fun and earn three times as much by being an accountant or a lawyer without taking on such onerous burdens?

Another criticism of deontological ethics is that the theory cannot resolve conflicts between the rights of different people, for example those of the mother and of the fetus in the rights-based approach to abortion discussed above. Duties may also conflict; for example, the duty of confidentiality may conflict with a duty of care for others, as with an epileptic who drives or a patient infected with human immunodeficiency virus (HIV) who will not tell his wife of his condition. There is the conflict between the duty of GPs in commissioning groups to obtain the best possible health care for the local population and the interpretation of the GMC's duty of the doctor to 'make the care of your patients your first concern' as meaning the patient in the consulting room. This is one example that is currently often discussed of how deontological thinking can be problematic in health care.

The consequentialist fragment

Moral theories that focus on trying to maximise the good, rather than on rights and duties, are known as consequentialist because they judge the rightness of actions by their consequences. If deontology is the fragment of moral discourse to which the GMC and professional bodies are clinging, then public health and its input into health policy and resource allocation seem to be attached to consequentialism. Because this theory considers the total sum of good that an action produces, irrespective of who benefits from it, it seems the ideal way to look at the health of populations. In the UK, health policies,[18] decisions by the National Institute for Health and Care Excellence (NICE) and the inclusion of activities in the GP Quality and Outcomes Framework (QOF) are often justified on grounds of 'health gain' – a consequentialist concept often measured in terms of QALYs – quality-adjusted life years.[19]

Although taken as axiomatic in these areas, consequentialism and QALYs are also widely criticised. It is suggested that QALYs further disadvantage the disadvantaged, because a life-extending intervention will add fewer QALYs to someone whose quality of life is already poor for some other reason than to someone otherwise in good health.[20] QALY-based analysis finds it hard to take account of individuality and different perceptions of the good. It has to assume that everyone shares the same consequentialist vision of the good. It also risks treating people as means rather than ends. If everyone with a high cholesterol takes a statin, we know how many heart attacks will be prevented in a population (assuming that the research data are valid and reliable) – but we have no means of knowing which individuals will avoid a heart attack, so a policy of promoting statin treatment for all at risk (such as the QOF) focuses on the good of the population as a whole rather than the choice of the individual.

Consequentialism cannot take account of the structure of an individual human narrative. In this view life is a series of episodes linked in an arbitrary manner; all that matters is the overall good of the episodes. When I was a child we used to play a game called 'Consequences' at Christmas. Pieces of paper were passed round, and each person added a line to a story, not knowing what went before or after. The resulting 'narrative' of who met whom, where, what they said and the consequence, was nonsensical, though often amusing. The consequentialist view of life is like this. The only sense that can be made of this meaningless tale is to maximise pleasurable episodes – to eat, drink and be merry.[21]

Because consequentialists emphasise the quantity of good in a life, rather than seeing it as a narrative with a purpose and shape, they have problems with its inevitable end in death. A philosophy that sees good as a longer and less painful life will naturally see death as something to be avoided for as long as possible. The postponement of death is of course doomed to failure (and often an expensive failure, as more and more resources are poured into resisting the inevitable) and society pays a high cost to support a long, slow decline by dementia and increased disability.[22] Conversely, however, when the pain of life outweighs its pleasure and will always do so, death is to be welcomed and indeed assisted. Thus consequentialist arguments are often used to support making elective death more easily available when the balance of good and suffering in a life becomes irreversibly negative.[23]

Other value-laden fragments

The two fragments I have discussed so far are traditional approaches to ethics. The incommensurable criticism each makes of the weaknesses of the other, which I have tried to summarise above, are well rehearsed in the moral philosophy literature. The other four fragments in our moral universe that I want to suggest are helpful in understanding the current state of confused moral discourse in medicine – legalism, managerialism, capitalism and consumerism – are less obviously ethical. Indeed they are often thought of as value free, but each of them in fact contains implicit values. As so often in health care because the values in these fragments are rarely explicit they are easily overlooked, and seen either as self-evident truths or statements of fact rather than evaluations.

These fragments are not totally separate; there are strong links between them and perhaps some of them might be better considered as one fragment rather than two – for example, are capitalism and consumerism different fragments, or two aspects of one conceptual framework that emphasise different aspects of it? This may be an interesting question but from the point of view of the purpose of this chapter, which is to establish whether MacIntyre's view that we live in a fragmented moral universe applies to health care, we only need to establish that such fragments exist and are incommensurable. It is not necessary to establish a definitive analysis of those fragments or the boundaries between them.

The legal fragment

If duty is the stern daughter of the voice of God, then the law is her even sterner granddaughter: a codification of rights and duties. The law takes suspicion as axiomatic, in a similar way that Descartes started from the premise that the only thing he could confidently believe was 'I think'.[24] In the law nothing is taken on trust, nothing believed without evidence. The Anglo-Saxon legal system in the UK has at its heart an adversarial relationship, since both civil and legal cases are tried by the two opposing parties each presenting their case. Although legalism derives its values from the law taken to extremes, its effect on health care cannot be blamed on lawyers. Lawyers may be free from legalism whilst non-lawyers may be extremely legalistic.

Legal frameworks for medical practice and health have existed in most times and places, but usually these set general boundaries, and within these limits professions were trusted to be self-governing, and much of the detail was left to the judgement of individual practitioners. Recently, however, legal and quasi-legal practices seem to have had a growing impact on medicine and health care. For example the GP Contract of 1947[25] defined the services that GPs were required to provide as 'those services usually provided by general practitioners'. This circular definition was replaced by a tighter contract in 2004,[26] in which many of those services were spelt out and the standards expected (and paid for) were defined in detail. Forty years ago the GMC policed doctors with a light touch, and so long as they avoided the 'Five As'[27] (Alcohol, Abortion, Adultery, Advertising and Association with non-licensed practitioners) it was assumed that their practice was satisfactory. Sadly medicine, like other professions, did not always justify this trust; doctors became 'a conspiracy against the laity',[28] banding together to conceal incompetence and impropriety. Those within the profession responsible for patrolling the boundaries of judgement and good practice often did not use the tools that existed to address inadequate performance. Too much was left to individual judgement, and the result was a series of catastrophes and scandals. As a result trust in the medical profession as a whole broke down for many politicians, managers and patient representatives, and multiple legal and quasi-legal procedures have been put in place to police the profession.[29] A naïve assumption that professionals are always to be trusted and respected by virtue of their position was replaced by a 'hermeneutic of suspicion'.[30] Consequently, rather than expecting that practitioners try to do their best and practise virtuously, this has to be proven regularly.

Another factor that may have contributed to the growth of legalism in medical practice is that our society, perhaps imbibing cultural norms from the United States, has become both more litigious[31] and more risk averse.[32] The latter stems in part from the former, because when legal challenge occurs the cost is enormous – in money, time and disruption. People therefore go to great lengths to avoid risk of litigation; placing as it were a 'fence around the law'. (This is an expression used of rabbinic laws (*gezeirah*), which are intended to protect Jews from violating a *mitzvah*, the commandments of the Torah, the Five Books of Moses in the Hebrew Bible. A classic example of building a fence around the Law relates to Exodus 23:19: 'You are not to boil a kid in the milk of its mother.' From this comes the rabbinical law that forbids mixing dairy products with meat in the same meal.[33])

This phenomenon is seen for example in health and safety[34] and data protection[35] where practice driven by fear often goes far beyond what the law actually requires. Health care involves both these issues and so is subject to these general social forces. Defensive practice is another example of risk aversion more specific to health care. Health professionals sometimes feel constrained to follow guidelines for fear of complaint or legal action, even if they are unconvinced of their relevance for a particular patient. This concern was for example expressed in a debate at the RCGP Annual Conference 2011 in Liverpool. In response to this, Prof. Sir Michael Rawlins, then Chair of NICE, pointed out that NICE issues guidelines, which as Sackett made clear need to be integrated with clinical judgement.[36] Sir Michael estimated that NICE guidelines would be applicable in perhaps 80% of cases; however, it is often assumed that they are protocols rather than guidelines, and that deviation from them always reflects substandard practice.

If at one time professions were a law unto themselves, 'conspiracies against the laity' banding together to conceal incompetence and impropriety, the pendulum seems now to have swung to the other extreme, so that multiple checks are in place, which take considerable time and money.[37] In GP training, rigorous documentation requirements[38] are driven by the need to be able to defend a judicial review of a decision to fail a student (and ideally make it clear to students who do fail that this is the case so that they don't even try), and the need to be able to defend a charge of contributory negligence in training a doctor who goes on to kill someone. The rather chilling view expressed by a respected teacher at my medical school – 'most of you will probably kill someone at some point. ... but that will be far outweighed by the number of lives you will save' – is no longer seen as an acceptable assessment of the balance of risks.

Managerialism

Having developed in the private sector, where effective management was seen to reduce costs and increase profits, management has in recent years gained a higher profile in the public and voluntary sector. Management is not an academic discipline or a philosophical framework; it is an eclectic collection of skills and techniques that can help organisations function better. Nor for the most part are its practices evidence-based in the sense clinical researchers would understand; robust research on managerial methods is surprisingly rare. Managerial initiatives are judged individually and empirically on their outcomes, and management texts tend to be narratives of success rather than reviews of controlled trials. This is not necessarily a bad thing – the same could be said of much medical practice, and there are many other sorts of evidence worth considering apart from randomised controlled trials – but it does perhaps mean that there are incommensurable ideas on the nature of evidence current in health care, which contributes to the moral confusion.

Good management has much to contribute to effective health care. Any activity needs good organisation and efficient administration if it is to be successful, and health care is no exception. But sometimes instead of being a means management becomes an end in itself; management becomes 'managerialism'. Edwards[39] suggests managerialism has four components: efficiency as the primary value guiding managers' actions and decisions; faith in the tools and techniques of management; a class consciousness among managers; and a view of managers as moral agents. Stephen Pattison calls this 'the faith of the managers'[40] and compares it to a fundamentalist religious faith.

As with lawyers and legalism, we must distinguish clearly between the role of managers and managerialism. Clinicians, particularly if they move into managerial roles within their profession, may imbibe, often unconsciously, the implicit values of managerialism – a change that may be recognised by colleagues – for example a GP who devoted an increasing amount of time to working with the Primary Care Trust was described to me as 'having gone over to the dark side'. And even clinicians with no particular management role may find their behaviour is influenced by their own 'inner managerialist'. Conversely managers may use the tools of management pragmatically to improve health care without having the values of managerialism.

The impact of managerialism on higher education was defined as 'the imposition of a powerful management body that overrides professional skills and knowledge. It keeps discipline under tight control and is driven by efficiency, external accountability and monitoring, and an emphasis on standards.'[41] Many health professionals will recognise this as describing a process that has increasingly affected their own professional lives in recent years.

Although management is essential, managerialism can have negative effects. Practitioners in social work,[42] higher education[43] and even the Church of England[44] as well as in health care have criticised its impact in their fields of work. So for example Philip Measure accuses social workers in management of becoming 'budget-obsessed/target-driven "clones" of the State'.[45] University lecturers feel that an

> intrusive culture means that people are not left to just get on with it in the way that they were. There is perhaps too much monitoring and too much written reporting … long hours packed with meetings, mountains of paperwork and email and the search for additional resources. Research was marginalised and there was little time for reflection.[46]

Because managerialism sees 'efficiency as the primary value guiding managers' actions and decisions'[47] and has 'faith in the tools and techniques of management' as the way to that efficiency, the processes of management become ends in themselves,[48] which some suggest can have a negative impact on morale and innovation. Cameron describes how he and colleagues set up an innovative treatment service for people with alcohol problems, driven by altruism and pride in the creation of a good service, but he sees such innovation as now impossible:

> I see managerialism as a virus which has as its main attribute the destruction of altruism and of individual clinical and scholarly activity. I think that is a bad thing, for it suppresses individual oddities like me. Managerialism does not allow outliers, but it is from those outliers, those mavericks, those oddballs that innovation is spawned. And I know that if the managerial systems we now live under in universities and the NHS existed 25 years ago, we would not have been able to do what we did.[49]

In medicine the values of managerialism may be seen as underlying hospital targets, such as the four-hour wait in Accident and Emergency Departments, the 18-week treatment targets[50], new to follow-up ratios, etc.[51] This may lead to an emphasis on what is most easily measured rather than what is perhaps most important. For example, some years ago I held the budget for a coronary prevention initiative in Inner London. Like most such projects we were adopting a multifactorial approach – working with GPs and other health professionals, but also taking part in initiatives to screen and educate people in other situations, for example shopping centres, community groups, etc. We were asked by those monitoring our grant for 'one outcome measure', and attempts to persuade them to accept multiple measures or a narrative review were unsuccessful.

The impact has perhaps been less in general practice than in hospitals because it is a more dispersed activity that is harder to control, and managers are often valued colleagues in small teams rather than distant figures demanding data and setting performance targets. Nevertheless its effect is still noticeable – most obviously in the impact of the QOF, but also in appraisal and the Performers

List. Those involved in GP training will be very aware of the ePortfolio,[52] which includes a number of managerial tools (360 degree appraisal, line-managers' reports, audits as well as large amounts of documentary evidence of performance). Revalidation has been implemented on the basis of faith in similar methods.[53]

There is no doubt an element of tribalism when there is tension between managers and professionals.[54] Some doctors do not respect genuine managerial expertise, and use clinical freedom as an excuse to avoid openness and accountability. Health service managers often come from nursing and other healthcare backgrounds whose relationship with medicine has sometimes been one of rivalry rather than collaboration. Managers do not have the lengthy training of clinicians, nor the high salaries and job security that this currently leads to in the UK. Although the contributions of clinicians and managers to good health care can be and often is complementary and amicable, these factors can produce remarkably aggressive class warfare. I have never felt such sustained antagonism as when I was the lone GP amongst a hundred nursing and health service managers at a Strategic Health Authority planning meeting. Relationships between academics, social workers or parish priests and their managers may perhaps involve similar stereotyping and tribal antagonisms. In deciding whether managerialism is a moral fragment that has an impact on the values of health care, it is important to put aside such prejudices. Managerialism is a value system that may be taken up by clinicians, politicians and the general public just as much as by managers.

Business and markets

Throughout most of the history of Western civilisation health care has been a mixture of a service provided for profit to those who could pay and a charitable act to those who could not. In Britain the latter was provided through monasteries and religious hospitals in the Middle Ages, and later through voluntary hospitals, but this provision was inevitably somewhat patchy. During the twentieth century in Europe[55] health care came to be seen as a basic service that a civilised and prosperous community should provide for all its members. Bismarck initiated the first social security system in Germany in 1889.[56] In the UK Lloyd George set up the National Insurance scheme for employed workers in 1911.[57] Conscription in the First World War revealed the poor health of much of the urban poor,[58] which led to the introduction of a variety of public health measures in the 1920s and 30s.[59] Finally in 1948 the National Health Service was set up, providing health care for all 'free at the point of use'.[60]

Initially, at a time when the merits of economic planning were more clearly seen than its disadvantages, the organisation of health care was based on a mixture of centralised planning and the well-meaning amateurism that had characterised earlier charitable systems. But as healthcare activity expanded (as it continually tends to do, with the development of new drugs and surgical procedures) costs rose. A universal taxation-funded health service means that when this happens then as taxpayers we all bear an increasing cost. There is thus a strong public interest in keeping down the cost of health care, just as there is equally a strong public interest in better health.

The most efficient healthcare systems in promoting health (in so far as this can be measured) tend to be those where financial systems like capitation payments[61] and gatekeeper systems[62] discourage unnecessary health care. But as the twentieth century drew to a close it became clear that this alone was not keeping costs under control.

The principle of universal, state-funded health care is now axiomatic in European culture, and we look with puzzlement at the United States where it is seen as radical. But although that principle was too deeply rooted to be challenged,[63] under the free-market economic policies pioneered by Margaret Thatcher and followed by her successors, market forces[64] came to be seen as the main drivers for efficiency and excellence. This view has been one reason for the growing impact of managerialism discussed above. Managerialism sees all activities, including education, religion and health care, as essentially businesses and therefore best managed using business methods.

But it has also led to a split between purchasers and providers, who are now seen as antagonists (in a similar adversarial way as in the law). Providers have an interest in increasing the provision of health care, whilst purchasers strive to keep costs down. From the market perspective health care is a service commodity, like restaurant meals or hotel accommodation. For healthcare professionals as providers the more health care you sell the better, and for patients as consumers the more you can purchase the better. In most areas of the market the consumer pays, but this is not so for health care, at least in Europe.

Markets are often thought of as value free; 'business is business' is a phrase often used to justify amoral if not immoral behaviour. But that does not mean that market thinking does not have implicit values. One of the central values of capitalism is that consumption is of itself a good thing, and the more goods and services you have the better for producer and consumer alike. Market methods have proved spectacularly successful at providing more goods and services. We have seen in the late twentieth century in Russia and Eastern Europe how ineffective economic planning is in this respect, and the superiority of free markets in encouraging growth is now generally accepted.

It has been argued that, above a certain level of absolute poverty, there may be no relationship between wealth and wellbeing;[65] you can become better off not by having more but by needing less.[66] Whether in general greater wealth necessarily means a better life is a question beyond the scope of this book, but it is surely true that more health care does not mean better health. Except perhaps for a few people with Münchausen syndrome or hypochondriasis health care is not an end in itself; rather it is a means to an end – that end being better health. Precisely what good health means will be discussed in Chapter 3, but however we define it, better health does not necessarily come from more health care.

Although as with wealth a certain minimum level of health care may be necessary for good health, there is a case to be made that, for a given state of health, the less health care we have the better. In this respect health care is akin to sanitary engineering; it is part of the underpinning of a good life, and like sanitary engineering when working well is unobtrusive and is best hidden. From a market perspective however the more goods there are to buy and sell the better for both consumer and provider.

The impact of these values in practice is complex and unpredictable. It is confounded by managerial targets, legal requirements, sets of rights and duties, and a public health commitment to maximising health gain. It does however mean that for a lot of the time the attention of people in health care is focused on issues some way away from health. Moreover market-driven healthcare systems consume more resources than planned systems, and the relationship between global health indicators and health expenditure is by no means linear.[67]

The consumerist fragment

Marxists might see the introduction of free health care as the effort of a ruling elite to maintain units of labour in good working order. Less cynical observers might think that political leaders felt an obligation to the poor based on altruistic, slightly paternalistic principles – a continuation of the longstanding tradition of charity to the poor and sick that from the Middle Ages onwards produced almshouses and charitable hospitals.[68] And, as in these institutions, for the most part people accepted what was offered and were grateful for it.

Whatever the motivation, in the early days of universal access to health and education, planning was used to ensure access to a service that was assumed to be of a similar (good) quality. Thus for example the Medical Practices Committee[69] regulated the number of GPs in each area so as to encourage an even distribution of GPs across the UK (in which it was highly successful – in contrast with many countries both rich and poor where doctors gravitate to the more attractive areas).[70] In doing this they did not enquire into what those GPs did or how effective it was.

In recent decades consumerism has become an increasingly powerful force in society; and more and more relationships are conceived in terms of customer and provider. Those who used trains and buses used to be passengers; those who rented a telephone line were subscribers. Now we are all 'customers'. Not everyone is happy with this concept:

> *I don't consume the bus when I ride, I'm a rider. I don't consume digital news, I learn and share it. I don't consume music, I listen, dance, and recommend. I'm not always a consumer.*[71]

When in the 1990s the market became a dominant way of thinking about health care, the split between purchasers and providers was visible to health professionals but it was not obvious to patients, who continued for the most part to attend their local GP and hospital as they had always done. More recently, however, building on the concept of health care as a market, consumerism has become a dominant mode of discourse in UK health care, and choice in public services has been emphasised, both as a patient entitlement and as a driver for service improvement.[72] The NHS Constitution,[73] which defines what users can expect from the NHS, is written very much as a customer's charter.

As a result we have a choice of providers. Commercial companies and walk-in centres[74] offer alternatives to traditional general practice. Hospitals are to be improved by offering patients the choice of where to go. The whole system is supported by computerised 'Choose and Book' software.[75] Despite its cost and technical problems an electronic booking system for hospital appointments has considerable advantages. Rather than the GP sending off a letter into the void in the hope that an appointment will be dispatched to the patient in due course (an act of faith that often felt similar to prayer!) the patient can leave the consultation with an appointment or the power to make one at a convenient time and be sure when and where they need to go. The risk of getting lost in the system, the letter going astray and no appointment being sent or sent to the wrong address is much diminished. But this has little to do with choice; indeed a system that offered the choice of a few local hospitals rather than providers throughout the UK might have been less costly and worked more rapidly. 'Choose' was added to 'Book' in the computer system because choice was seen as good in itself, and as a lever to drive up quality through competition.

Consumerism is a rationalist model, in which the rational consumer makes a free and informed choice of goods on offer, but if the information is not available on which to make choices rationally they are little more than gambles. Most patients choose to go either to the nearest hospital or to one reasonably nearby where they will be seen most quickly.[76] Sophisticated judgements on quality of care are rare, because in health care few people actually have the information to make judgements on quality. Thus in a Department of Health survey the main reason patients gave for making their choice was (quite sensibly) cleanliness and low infection rates[77] but in reality how many patients (or even GPs?) have this information to hand when making their choices? It may be that, for the vast majority of patients, choice is a chimera.[78]

Where people do have strong preferences these are often based on hearsay or anecdotal experience, or fuelled by irrational prejudices. Patients may refuse to see a cardiologist as an out-patient at a certain hospital because an elderly relative had a bad experience of the nursing on a geriatric ward, or died following surgery there. Even general practitioners, with greater familiarity with individual practitioners and a better understanding of what contributes to high-quality care, are often only able to advise on the basis of a general impression of performance based on a small and probably unrepresentative sample.

Many of the same problems apply to other areas of health care. As with any specialist service, ignorance amongst users inhibits the operation of market forces. The consumer is not in a position to assess the quality of the product, or even if they need it at all. Therefore the customer is forced to judge on the basis of peripherals – whether the organisation is smart and efficient, whether the staff are friendly – which may or may not correlate with technical ability. Also many crucial aspects of health care are very private – they take place in the consulting room, with only the clinician and the patient present.

These are empirical problems with a consumerist approach to health care. But there are also evaluative issues. Choice tends to favour convenience over continuity, in the belief that 'customers' used to shopping at any time and with no notice value similar convenience in accessing general practice and other aspects of health care. Initiatives such as advanced access[79] and extended GP hours[80] have been promoted to make this easier. And if it is still not convenient to see your general practitioner then walk-in centres and minor injury units provide alternative 'choices'. But such choices make it harder to develop and sustain personal relationships between patients and clinicians over time.

From the consumerist perspective this doesn't matter, because health care is seen as an impersonally provided service. It doesn't really matter whether I get my groceries from Sainsbury's or Tesco; both are large anonymous organisations with which it is impossible to have a personal relationship; quality is assured by managerial systems rather than on the basis of trust in an individual, as it might be with a small shopkeeper. From the consumerist perspective health care is seen as like this; it's value for money and reliability of the product rather than a relationship with the provider that matters. One consequence of this model is that pharmacy services, which used to be provided mostly by individuals working alone, are now mostly provided by chains and supermarkets.[81] But many people would argue that in health care relationships do matter. One clinician, be she doctor, nurse or pharmacist, who sees a patient regularly, can get a better grasp of complex problems than is possible in a succession of one-off encounters. And of course often the relationship itself is a central part of the therapy.[82]

Another important issue of values is that the first priority of the doctor in a consumerist model is not to mend the patient's broken body-machine, to help her understand her illness or to keep her healthy, but to keep her happy. In consumerism the customer is always right. At first sight this does not seen unreasonable; after all, health care exists to benefit the patient rather than the doctor. Should not patients decide what they want out of general practice, rather than doctors deciding paternalistically for them? But there are situations where this view raises problems. General practitioners are often approached by people who request drugs of addiction, often on some improbable pretext. Consumerism implies that the doctor should accede to this request, but a doctor who does this would be considered a bad doctor by colleagues, and by the general public outside the subculture of addictive drug use. Indeed in extreme cases this is one reason for a doctor being removed from the medical list.[83]

In less extreme cases than this general practitioners are often asked for something that in their view is not for the best. Patients with back pain commonly ask for an X-ray, believing that this will shed light on the situation; in fact it rarely helps and exposes the patient to unnecessary, potentially harmful radiation.[84] Do we want a consumerism where the doctor accedes to such requests? An alternative view is that the patient looks for and directly or indirectly pays for an expert opinion. If a shopping analogy is appropriate, it is perhaps the specialist shopkeeper who advises customers on sound purchases within a narrow range of goods that is the parallel, not the 'pile them high and sell them cheap' self-service hypermarket.

Consumerism, like legalism, is an adversarial model that pits patient against professionals in a battle of wits. Unlike legalism however its emphasis on choice and competition also puts professionals at odds with each other as commercial rivals.

Consumerism has risen alongside the rise in concern for patient autonomy in medical ethics, though which is cause and which is effect is not clear. Seeing patients as rational consumers is one way to safeguard their autonomy, but the link is perhaps contingent rather than necessary. Perhaps there are bases other than consumerism for the belief that patients should be empowered to make decisions about health and the health service, and particularly about their own health care?

Tensions and conflicts between the fragments

These six fragments are just one way of looking at the perspectives we take on values in health care; there may be other analyses that give us a better understanding of the situation we face. It does however seem credible on the basis of this analysis that health care is conducted in a climate where there are conceptual fragments with different value structures, as MacIntyre suggests. If he is right then we should also be able to find situations where these fragments conflict and lead to incommensurable conflicts in values.

The relationship between these fragments is complicated. Sometimes they share values with each other and work together. Sometimes they pull in different directions, threatening to tear the fabric of health care apart. But there do seem to be problems in trying to use all of them together. Consumerism places emphasis on convenience, choice and individual autonomy, but these are incompatible with a public health policy that seeks to maximise the corporate good. This tension was for example seen recently in the debate about the merits of rewarding general practitioners for offering extended opening hours rather than using the resources on other more clinical activities.[85]

The foundation of professionalism is trust,[86] but the basis of legalism, consumerism and markets is suspicion; all cast doctor and patient in adversarial roles. Perhaps because of this adversarial position, the tension between autonomy and paternalism, a central issue in medical ethics for the last generation, remains fundamentally unresolved. This contributes to the breakdown in the trust fundamental to relationships between professionals and their clients.

Also because our moral values and frameworks are so often unconscious it is common to find people as it were standing on two disconnected moral fragments, a position that can be uncomfortable when they start drifting apart, as anyone who has stood with one foot in a boat and the other on the bank will know. We see this for example in the NHS, whose constitution is deontology tinged with consumerism, but whose budget allocation system is consequentialist.

Managerialism is often combined with the suspicion and risk aversion that comes from legalism. Hilton[87] describes how this process affected audit of companies by accountants:

When accounting and auditing standards were first introduced in the 1970's in response to a series of accounting scandals they were resisted by some on the grounds that accountancy was a profession and the whole point of a profession was to deliver a considered judgement on complex issues. Society had invented professions to provide guidance when there was no clearly right answer.

He says these sceptics predicted that within a generation judgement would be eroded until audit was seen as a useless, box-ticking exercise, and argues that we have now reached that point and calls for a return to professional judgement in auditing. QOF leads and GP trainers may feel that health care is heading down the same road to futility.

Consultations that doctors find difficult often involve a collision between moral fragments. Consider this scenario: a patient comes in convinced that he needs an antibiotic for a sore throat, otitis media or chest infection, sleeping tablets or strong, addictive opioid painkillers, and is not open to a discussion of the pros and cons of this and other options.

Such patients are clinging to a consumerist fragment; they are the customer and the customer is always right. If the doctor does not provide the service requested he is 'patronising' or 'arrogant' (words used of me in complaints that revealed these values). A doctor in this situation clings to a legalistic or consequentialist fragment (I am following the rules of good practice, and/or doing what in most cases would lead to the best outcome for the patient). Encounters like this do not help either doctor or patient to flourish.

A different type of problem occurs when the patient comes with a problem that she wants to talk about, but the doctor, driven by the pressure of the QOF, wants to talk about smoking, measure the blood pressure and check the weight. Many doctors and patients feel that this consequentialist agenda gets in the way of what they want to achieve.

What should we do?

As a philosopher MacIntyre is concerned about the 'incommensurability of moral discourse'.[88] He wants a coherent, unified and logical moral framework. To pragmatic clinicians, used to picking up conceptual tools and using them without worrying too much about theoretical foundations or logical coherence, this may seem an academic concern far removed from the realities of clinical practice. Many of the problems health care faces are practical, and the inconsistencies that I have pointed out may not seem particularly relevant to their solution. Yet MacIntyre is not merely concerned about the fragmentation of moral discourse because it is intellectually untidy; he argues that it leads to a fragmentation of human life and a deep-seated dissatisfaction and *anomie*. If we are to progress in the search for the good life, he argues, then we need to overcome this fragmentation.

He suggests the solution is a form of virtue ethics radically different from conventional deontology and utilitarianism. Is it possible to produce a MacIntyrean model of healthcare ethics based on his ideas? What are its potential benefits? Will this help us deal with the practical as well as the conceptual problems we face? This question will be considered in the next chapter.

Notes

1. MacIntyre A. *After Virtue* (2nd edn). London: Duckworth, 1985.

2. MacIntyre. *After Virtue*, p. 1.

3. Pope John Paul II. *Evangelium Vitae: encyclical on the value and inviolability of human life.* 1995. www.catholic-pages.com/documents/evangelium_vitae.pdf [accessed 4 March 2014].

4. McMahan J. The right to choose an abortion. *Philosophy and Public Affairs* 1993; **22(4)**: 331–48.

5. Thompson JJ. A defense of abortion (from *Philosophy and Public Affairs* 1971; **1(1)**), reprinted in R Munson (ed.), *Intervention and Reflection: basic issues in medical ethics* (5th edn). Belmont: Wadsworth, 1996, pp. 69–80, http://spot.colorado.edu/~heathwoo/Phil160,Fall02/thomson.htm [accessed 16 January 2014].

6. Fagan A. Human rights. In: *Internet Encyclopaedia of Philosophy.* 2005. www.iep.utm.edu/hum-rts/#SH3b [accessed 16 January 2014].

7. United Nations. The universal declaration of human rights, article 26, www.un.org/en/documents/udhr/index.shtml [accessed 16 January 2014].

8. Harrison R. Jeremy Bentham. In: T Honderich (ed.), *The Oxford Companion to Philosophy.* Oxford: Oxford University Press, 1995, pp. 85–8, www.utilitarian.net/bentham/about/1995----.htm [accessed 16 January 2014].

9. Human Rights Act 1998. www.legislation.gov.uk/ukpga/1998/42/contents [accessed 16 January 2014].

10. Department of Health. *The NHS Constitution.* London: DH, 2010, http://webarchive.nationalarchives.gov.uk/20130107105354/http://www.dh.gov.uk/en/Publicationsandstatistics/Publications/PublicationsPolicyAndGuidance/DH_113613 [accessed 16 January 2014].

11. Evans HM. Do patients have duties? *Journal of Medical Ethics* 2007; **33(12)**: 689–94.

12. General Medical Council. Duties of a doctor: the duties of a doctor registered with the General Medical Council. In: *Good Medical Practice.* London: GMC, 2013, www.gmc-uk.org/guidance/good_medical_practice/duties_of_a_doctor.asp [accessed 16 January 2014].

13. Health Professions Council. *Standards of Conduct, Performance and Ethics.* London: HPC, 2008, www.hpc-uk.org/assets/documents/10002367FINALcopyofSCPEJuly2008.pdf [accessed 16 January 2014].

14. Nursing and Midwifery Council. *The Code: standards of conduct, performance and ethics.* London: NWC, 2008, www.nmc-uk.org/Nurses-and-midwives/Standards-and-guidance1/The-code/The-code-in-full/ [accessed 16 January 2014].

15. Dicker A. Obligations of general practitioners to substance misusers. *Journal of the Royal Society of Medicine* 1999; **92(8)**: 422–4.

16. William Wordsworth, 'Ode to Duty', line 1, www.poetry-archive.com/w/ode_to_duty.html [accessed 16 January 2014].

17. Skinner C. Kant on acting from duty and acting in accordance with duty. 2011. http://askaphilosopher.wordpress.com/2011/07/22/kant-on-acting-from-duty-and-acting-in-accordance-with-duty/ [accessed 16 January 2014].

18. National Institute for Health and Care Excellence. Measuring effectiveness and cost effectiveness: the QALY. 2010. www.nice.org.uk/newsroom/features/measuringeffectivenessandcosteffectivenesstheqaly.jsp [accessed 16 January 2014].

19. Phillips C, Thompson G. *What is a QALY?* London: Hayward Medical Communications, 2001, www.medicine.ox.ac.uk/bandolier/painres/download/whatis/QALY.pdf [accessed 16 January 2014].

20. Harris J. QALYfying the value of human life. *Journal of Medical Ethics* 1987; **13(3)**: 117–23.

21. Ecclesiastes 8: 15.

22. Mangin D, Sweeney K, Heath I. Preventive health care in elderly people needs rethinking *British Medical Journal* 2007; **335**: 285, www.bmj.com/content/335/7614/285 [accessed 16 January 2014].

23. Glover J. *Causing Death and Saving Life*. Harmondsworth: Penguin, 1977.

24. Descartes R. *Discours de la Méthode*. Paris: Maxi Poche, 1995 [1637] and many other editions.

25. National Health Service. *General Medical Services Statutory Instrument No. 635*. London: HMSO, 1992.

26. Rivett G. 1997–2008 Labour's decade. In: *National Health Service History*. www.nhshistory.net/chapter_6.html#Contractual discussions [accessed 16 January 2014].

27. Smith T. The parliamentary scene: struck off. *Journal of Medical Ethics* 1981; **7**: 212.

28. Shaw GB. *The Doctor's Dilemma*. London: Penguin, 1946 [1911].

29. Skeggs J. A critical analysis of the multiple performance management processes for dealing with cases of sexual misconduct by general practitioners in the UK. Dissertation submitted in part fulfilment of an MSc in Primary Care, Queen Mary University of London, 2010.

30. Atkins K. Paul Ricoeur (1913–2005). In: *Internet Encyclopaedia of Philosophy*. www.iep.utm.edu/ricoeur [accessed 16 January 2014].

31. Chacko D. Medical liability litigation: an historical look at the causes for its growth in the United Kingdom. In: Esteves LR, Gardner L (eds), *University of Oxford Discussion Papers in Economic and Social History*. 2009. www.nuff.ox.ac.uk/economics/history/Paper77/77chacko.pdf [accessed 16 January 2014].

32. Neuberger J. *Unkind, Risk Averse and Untrusting: if this is today's society, can we change it?* York: Joseph Rowntree Foundation, 2008 www.jrf.org.uk/publications/unkind-risk-averse-and-untrusting-if-todays-society-can-we-change-it [accessed 16 January 2014].

33. Judaism 101, www.jewfaq.org/halakhah.htm [accessed 16 January 2014].

34. Health and Safety Executive. Myth: health and safety has gone mad! 2010. www.hse.gov.uk/myth/dec10.htm [accessed 16 January 2014].

35. Whitehead J. Photography and filming in school: when the Data Protection Act applies. Protecting Children Update. 2007. www.optimus-education.com/photography-and-filming-school-when-data-protection-act-applies [accessed 16 January 2014].

36. Sackett DL, Rosenberg WM, Gray JA, *et al*. Evidence based medicine: what it is and what it isn't. *British Medical Journal* 1996; **312(7023)**: 71–2, www.ncbi.nlm.nih.gov/pmc/articles/PMC2349778/pdf/bmj00524-0009.pdf [accessed 16 January 2014].

37. Skeggs. A critical analysis (*op. cit.*).

38. Stillman K. A service evaluation of the nMRCGP e-portfolio learning log as an educational tool for developing reflexive practice in GP trainees. Dissertation submitted in part fulfilment of an MA, University of the South Bank, 2012.

39. Edwards JD. Managerial influences in public administration. University of Tennessee Master of Public Administration materials. www.utc.edu/Academic/MasterofPublicAdministration/managerialism.htm [16 January 2014].

40. Pattison S. *The Faith of the Managers*. London: Cassell, 1997.

41. Outbreak of 'new managerialism' infects faculties. *Times Higher Education Supplement*, 2001, www.timeshighereducation.co.uk/story.asp?storyCode=164003&sectioncode=26 [accessed 16 January 2014].

42. Philip Measure accuses social workers in management becoming 'budget-obsessed/target-driven "clones" of the State'. The Social Care Experts Blog, 6 March 2008, www.communitycare.co.uk/blogs/social-care-experts-blog/2008/03/service-users-and-social-care.html [accessed 16 January 2014].

43. Outbreak of 'new managerialism' infects faculties (*op. cit.*).

44. Lewis-Anthony J. Fees, managerialism and the death of the Church of England. *Guardian*, 8 July 2011, www.guardian.co.uk/commentisfree/belief/2011/jul/08/church-of-england-parish-fees-orders [accessed 16 January 2014].

45. Philip Measure accuses social workers in management becoming 'budget-obsessed/target-driven "clones" of the State' (*op. cit.*).

46. Outbreak of 'new managerialism' infects faculties (*op. cit*).

47. Edwards JD. Managerial influences in public administration (*op. cit*).

48. *Yes Minister* and *Yes Prime Minister*. BBC Comedy, www.bbc.co.uk/comedy/yesminister/ [accessed 16 January 2014].

49. Cameron D. I see managerialism as a virus. *Guardian*, 4 April 2002, www.guardian.co.uk/society/2002/apr/05/publicvoices4 [accessed 16 January 2014].

50. NHS Choices. Waiting times. 2011. www.nhs.uk/choiceintheNHS/Rightsandpledges/Waitingtimes/Pages/Guide%20to%20waiting%20times.aspx [accessed 16 January 2014].

51. NHS. Outpatients – new to follow up ratios. 2008. www.improvement.nhs.uk/heart/sustainability/outpatients/new.html [25 March 2013].

52. RCGP Trainee ePortfolio. https://gpeportfolio.rcgp.org.uk/Login.aspx [accessed 16 January 2014].

53. General Medical Council. *The Good Medical Practice Framework for Appraisal and Revalidation*. London: GMC, 2011, www.gmc-uk.org/doctors/revalidation/revalidation_gmp_framework.asp [accessed 16 January 2014].

54. Kennedy I. The complexity of culture. In: *The Report of the Public Inquiry into Children's Heart Surgery at the Bristol Royal Infirmary 1984–1995: learning from Bristol*. London: DH, 2001, § 3, http://webarchive.nationalarchives.gov.uk/+/www.dh.gov.uk/en/Publicationsandstatistics/Publications/PublicationsPolicyAndGuidance/DH_4005620 [accessed 16 January 2014].

55. Jakubowski E, Busse R. *Health Care Systems in the EU: a comparative study* (European Parliament Directorate General for Research Working Paper). Luxembourg: European Parliament, www.europarl.europa.eu/workingpapers/saco/pdf/101_en.pdf [accessed 16 January 2014].

56. Social Security history: Otto von Bismarck. US Government, Social Security online. www.ssa.gov/history/ottob.html [accessed 16 January 2014].

57. Blake RNW, *et al.* David Lloyd George. *Encyclopaedia Britannica*, www.britannica.com/EBchecked/topic/345191/David-Lloyd-George [accessed 16 January 2014].

58. Winter JM. Military fitness and civilian health in Britain during the First World War. *Journal of Contemporary History* 1980; **15(2)**: 211–44, www.jstor.org/stable/260511 [accessed 16 January 2014].

59. Gorsky M. Public health in interwar England and Wales: did it fail? *Dynamis* 2008; **28**: 175–98, www.ncbi.nlm.nih.gov/pmc/articles/PMC2647660/ [accessed 16 January 2014].

60. NHS Choices. About the National Health Service (NHS). www.nhs.uk/NHSEngland/thenhs/about/Pages/overview.aspx [accessed 16 January 2014].

61. Rice N, Smith P. *Approaches to Capitation and Risk Adjustment in Health Care: an international survey.* York: Centre for Health Economics, University of York, 1999, www.york.ac.uk/che/pdf/op38.pdf [accessed 16 January 2014].

62. Mathers N, Hodgkin P. The Gatekeeper and the Wizard: a fairy tale. *British Medical Journal* 1989; **298(6667)**: 172–4, www.ncbi.nlm.nih.gov/pmc/articles/PMC1835499/ [accessed 16 January 2014].

63. Rivett G. 1978–1987 Clinical advance and financial crisis. In: *National Health Service History.* www.nhshistory.net/chapter_4.htm [accessed 16 January 2014].

64. Rivett G. 1988–1997 New influences and new pathways. In: *National Health Service History.* www.nhshistory.net/chapter_5.htm#The NHSreview [accessed 16 January 2014].

65. Staff writer. Happiness is ... 'gross national happiness' trumps GNP. *NYR Natural News*, 10 April 2012, www.nyrnaturalnews.com/health/2012/04/happiness-is-gross-national-happiness-trumps-gnp [accessed 16 January 2014].

66. Maitland S. *A Book of Silence.* London: Granta, 2008.

67. World Health Organization. *World Health Statistics 2010.* Geneva: WHO, www.who.int/whosis/whostat/2010/en/index.html [accessed 16 January 2014].

68. Manco J. Heritage of mercy. *Medieval History*, November 2003, www.buildinghistory.org/articles/heritagemercy.shtml [accessed 16 January 2014].

69. The Medical Practices Committee. http://webarchive.nationalarchives.gov.uk/+/www.dh.gov.uk/ab/Archive/MPC/index.htm [accessed 16 January 2014].

70. World Health Organization. *Increasing Access to Health Workers in Remote and Rural Areas through Improved Retention.* Background paper for the first expert meeting to develop evidence-based recommendations to increase access to health workers in remote and rural areas through improved retention (draft). Geneva: WHO, 2009, www.who.int/hrh/migration/background_paper.pdf [accessed 16 January 2014].

71. Comment on the overuse of the term consumer posted by 'Judic', 8 April 2010, www.consumerchoice.org [accessed 16 January 2014].

72. Department of Health. *Creating a Patient-Led NHS: delivering the NHS Improvement Plan.* London: DH, 2005, http://webarchive.nationalarchives.gov.uk/+/www.dh.gov.uk/en/publicationsandstatistics/publications/publicationspolicyandguidance/dh_4106506 [accessed 16 January 2014].

73. Department of Health. *NHS Constitution Interactive Version 2012*. www.nhs.uk/
    choiceintheNHS/Rightsandpledges/NHSConstitution/Documents/nhs-constitution-
    interactive-version-march-2012.pdf [accessed 16 January 2014].

74. NHS Emergency and urgent care services: walk-in centres. 2013. www.nhs.uk/
    NHSEngland/AboutNHSservices/Emergencyandurgentcareservices/pages/Walk-
    incentresSummary.aspx [accessed 16 January 2014].

75. Welcome to Choose and Book. 2012. www.chooseandbook.nhs.uk [accessed 16 January
    2014].

76. Dixon A, ApplebyJ, Robertson R, *et al*. *Patient Choice: how patients choose and how providers
    respond*. London: DH, 2010, www.kingsfund.org.uk/current_projects/patient_choice
    [accessed 16 January 2014].

77. Dixon S. *Report of the National Patient Choice Survey: September 2008 England*. London: DH,
    2009, webarchive.nationalarchives.gov.uk/20130107105354/http://www.dh.gov.uk/en/
    Publicationsandstatistics/Publications/PublicationsStatistics/DH_094013 [accessed 16
    January 2014].

78. Jones L, Mays N. *Systematic Review of the Impact of Patient Choice of Provider in the English
    NHS*. London: School of Hygiene and Tropical Medicine, 2009, http://hrep.lshtm.ac.uk/
    publications/Choice%20review%20March%202009.pdf [accessed 16 January 2014].

79. National Institute for Health Research. An evaluation of approaches to improving access
    to general practitioner appointments. 2008. www.nets.nihr.ac.uk/__data/assets/pdf_
    file/0017/81341/RS-08-1310-070.pdf [accessed 4 March 2014].

80. Campbell J. Access to primary care: advanced ... or smart? *British Journal of General
    Practice* 2007; **57(541)**: 603–4.

81. Taylor D. The apothecary's return? A brief look at pharmacy's future. In: S Anderson
    (ed.), *Making Medicines: a history of pharmacy and pharmaceuticals*. London: Pharmaceutical
    Press, 2005, pp. 283–99, www.pharmpress.com/files/docs/samplechapter05.pdf
    [accessed 16 January 2014].

82. Balint M. *The Doctor, His Patient and the Illness* (2nd edn). London: Churchill Livingstone,
    1964 [1957].

83. Ryder doctor struck off. *BBC News*, 11 December 2002, http://news.bbc.co.uk/1/hi/
    entertainment/2564911.stm [accessed 16 January 2014].

84. Kerry S, Hilton S, Patel S, *et al*. Routine referral for radiography of patients presenting
    with low back pain: is patients' outcome influenced by GPs' referral for plain radiography?
    Health Technology Assessment 2000; **4(20)**, www.hta.ac.uk/fullmono/mon420.pdf [accessed
    16 January 2014].

85. Longer GP opening hours branded wasteful 'PR exercise' by doctors. *Scotsman*,
    12 March 2009, www.scotsman.com/news/longer-gp-opening-hours-branded-wasteful-
    pr-exercise-by-doctors-1-1029586# [accessed 16 January 2014].

86. Koehn D. *The Ground of Professional Ethics*. London: Routledge, 1994.

87. Hilton A. *Evening Standard*, 6 July 2011, p. 28.

88. MacIntyre. *After Virtue* (*op. cit*).

Chapter 2

The practice of health care

I hope that in the last chapter I have shown how MacIntyre's analysis is helpful in understanding some of the disquiet in health care today. But Kuhn[1] pointed out that evidence that a theory is not working is insufficient to start a scientific revolution; a credible alternative is needed. In a similar way an analysis of fragmentation cannot provoke moral reform; people need to sight a lifeboat before they can abandon the philosophical flotsam to which they are clinging. In this chapter the attempt to construct the lifeboat, or rather customise one for health care from a kit designed by Alasdair MacIntyre, begins.

The lifeboat kit

MacIntyre[2] suggests that we need a system that is not just an intellectual theory of morality or even a set of desirable personal characteristics or virtues, but also a social structure to which the pursuit of virtue, both for its own sake and as a means to the construction of flourishing life narratives, is central. In this respect MacIntyre's approach differs from accounts of virtues in medical practice like those of Pellegrino and Thomasma,[3,4] which emphasise the importance of personal qualities in ensuring good clinical practice but neglect their contribution to the wellbeing of the moral agent: a deontology with a holistic concept of human character rather than a virtue ethic focused on *eudaemonia*.

In the moral tradition of Aristotle,[5] Aquinas[6] and MacIntyre, teleology, virtue and *eudaemonia* (the good life, the life worth living) are indissolubly interlinked. Life has a purpose or *telos*; virtues are qualities we need to achieve that purpose, and *eudaemonia* is the life story which achieves that purpose and is one in which the virtues are consistently demonstrated. MacIntyre anchors this link firmly in the structure of society. He defines a virtue as 'an acquired human quality, the possession and exercise of which tends to enable us to achieve those goods which are internal to practices, and the lack of which effectively prevents us from achieving any such goods'.[7] This definition depends on the specific meaning that he gives to the terms *practice* and *internal goods*.

Practices

He defines a practice as:

any coherent and complex form of socially established cooperative human activity through which goods internal to that form of activity are realised in the course of trying to achieve those standards of excellence which are appropriate to, and partially definitive of, that form of activity, with the result that human powers to achieve excellence, and human conceptions of the ends and goods involved, are systematically extended.[8]

Practices are complex – they are 'never just a set of technical skills', although 'every practice does require the exercise of technical skills'.[9] Rather, skills are a means to the end of practices, which is that the 'conceptions of the relevant goods and ends which the technical skills serve … are transformed and enriched by these extensions of human powers and by that regard for its own internal goods'.[10]

Although MacIntyre's system is fundamentally a virtue ethic, he does not completely abandon rules – practice 'involves standards of excellence and obedience to rules as well as the achievement of goods'.[11] Standards of excellence imply that it makes sense to say that someone is a good footballer, chemist, musician or farmer. We may debate precisely what it means to be a good X-er, but if X is a practice this is a meaningful concept. Participation in a practice involves trying to achieve those standards of excellence to the best of one's ability. I shall consider what those standards of excellence might be in relation to health and illness in Chapters 3 and 4, whilst Chapter 5 and 6 will deal with the qualities practitioners need to achieve those standards of excellence, and Chapter 7 explores the institutions that support them.

Practices have rules and standards (more or less arbitrary and more or less explicit) that must be obeyed – 'we cannot be initiated into a practice without accepting the authority of the best standards realised so far.'[12] But they are not static – 'the standards are not themselves immune from criticism' so 'practices never have a goal or goals fixed for all time' and 'the goals themselves are transmuted by the history of the activity'.[13] Practices are cooperative. Even if a practice necessarily involves solitary activity – for example painting, or scientific research – these things are taught and the people involved discuss, argue about, and often develop them together. A practice has an identifiable history (perhaps better thought of as a tradition), so that 'to enter into a practice is to enter into a relationship not only with its contemporary practitioners, but also with those who have preceded us in the practice, particularly those whose achievements extended the reach of the practice to its present point.'[14]

Internal and external goods

The other central concept in MacIntyre's theory is a distinction between internal and external goods. These differ in two important characteristics. First, 'it is characteristic of external goods that when achieved they are always some individual's property and possession' and 'characteristically they are such that the more someone has of them the less there is for other people'.[15] External goods are 'characteristically objects of competition'[16] in which there must be losers as well as winners. This obviously includes material goods such as money and other possessions gained through practices, but also some non-material goods that have these characteristics, such as fame and power. In contrast, although internal goods are 'the outcome of competition to excel' it is characteristic of them that 'their achievement is a good for the whole community who participate in the practice'[17] and their possession by one person does not take them away from another – indeed it enriches them. Knowledge, happiness and love are internal goods. If you teach me something then knowledge is increased, because I know it but you still know it too. One person's happiness does not diminish another's – indeed it often increases it (think of the experience of watching children play, for example). Internal goods (unlike external goods, or energy or mass) are not subject to any law of conservation.

MacIntyre argues that, unlike external goods, internal goods are unique to particular practices, and their value can only be fully appreciated by participating wholeheartedly in the relevant practice in a sincere attempt to achieve excellence according to the rules (explicit or implicit) of the practice. In contrast the link between external goods like money, power or prestige and a practice is a matter of social custom, not of necessity, and they can be achieved through a practice irrespective of how one participates in it. The same external goods can come through many practices, and may be obtained whatever degree of commitment is put into it; indeed cynics would argue that another characteristic of external goods is that they are unrelated to the excellence of the practitioner.

MacIntyre's example[18] is of a child bribed to play chess by the promise of sweets if she wins. The sweets are external goods, whilst the pleasure that derives from playing chess well – 'the achievement of a certain highly particular kind of analytic skill, strategic imagination and competitive intensity'[19] – is a good internal to the practice. So long as the child only plays to get the sweets, it does not matter to her whether she cheats or not, so long as she wins. Cheating however renders unattainable the internal goods of chess, the satisfaction of exercising that analytic skill and strategic imagination uniquely developed and obtained through chess.

Miller[20] points out that MacIntyre drew many of his examples and much of his thinking on practices from activities like chess, other games and the fine arts, which exist solely for their own sake – in MacIntyrean terminology for the sake of the internal goods achieved by participants and the contemplation of those goods by others. These Miller calls 'self-contained' practices. He suggests that there is another category of practices that exist to serve social ends beyond themselves, which he calls 'purposive practices'. These are commonly means through which people earn their living. Architecture is a good example. Although the need to earn a living (an external good in MacIntyre's nomenclature) may be the initial reason why an individual participates in that practice and is not for example a sculptor or a full-time chess player, earning a living is not the only good that comes from being an architect. If an architect is to be fulfilled in his profession he must enjoy his work and get satisfaction from it – part of which comes from doing it as well as possible.

Is health care a practice?

There can be few socially established human activities of which the words practice and practitioner are so widely used as medicine, although MacIntyre himself is ambiguous on its status as a practice. He uses medicine as an example of a practice in *After Virtue*, but earlier[21] he suggested that our moral confusion is so great that the only way to deal with it is for each doctor to advertise her moral principles as she advertises her opening hours and scales of charges. This indicates his pessimism on the coherence of medicine as a functioning practice in society today.

Is this pessimism justified? Despite the moral fragmentation explored in Chapter 1, medicine (at least in the UK and the rest of Europe) still has many of the characteristics that MacIntyre attributes to a practice. It is a complex socially established human activity; *ars longa, vita brevis* (the Latin translation more commonly used in the West than either the English 'art is long, life is short'[22] or Hippocrates' original Greek). It has a history in Western culture that stretches without a break to Hippocrates, in both its practical knowledge and its ethical standards. This tradition continues to influence practitioners,[23] though it may have been challenged and distorted by the post-Enlightenment moral fragmentation, and perhaps more recently by the influence of the fragments discussed in the last chapter and an emphasis on 'modernisation'[24] and up-to-date practice,[25] which can be linked to a lack of respect for tradition and denigration of the contribution of past practitioners.

Health care is not just a technical skill, although it involves the exercise of many such skills by a variety of practitioners. Although impaired by the fragmented moral framework discussed above it retains sufficient coherence to be recognised as a cooperative activity, albeit perhaps a rather confused one. It certainly has both explicit and implicit rules. It is taught and endlessly discussed, argued about and developed amongst its practitioners, and equally by people in general, from documentaries in the media to conversations on buses.

Although the rise of legalism and managerialism have made it more impersonal, the training of doctors and nurses is still basically an apprenticeship in which the would-be practitioner enters into a relationship with contemporary practitioners and has to accept the authority of recognised standards of excellence and obey received rules. And the established practitioner may expand and develop the tradition by challenging and modifying those rules, although as suggested in Chapter 1 legalism and managerialism may have made this harder.[26] Despite the difficulties in defining the good practitioner, no one argues that this is a meaningless question, and virtue continues to play a part in thinking about health care. So perhaps health care is a distorted rather than a destroyed practice.

The practice of medicine or the practice of health care?

Both MacIntyre and Miller talk of medicine rather than health care, perhaps because conventionally we refer to doctors as 'practising' medicine, but less often refer to nurses or physiotherapists practising their professions. Or perhaps to those outside health care it is incorrectly seen as synonymous with the work of doctors, and nurses along with other health professionals, managers and administrators are seen as playing subsidiary, supporting roles.

Whatever the reason, the brief discussions of MacIntyre and Miller of medicine as a practice suggest that it is one in which only doctors and possibly by extension other health professionals engage. But let us try a 'thought experiment'. If a Martian anthropologist were to arrive in our hospitals and health centres to study the complex socially established cooperative human activity going on there she would quite soon identify two distinct roles. Some ('professionals') would come and go regularly over long periods, staying for a large part of the day – a pattern of activity she observed in other contexts and called 'going to work'. If she were very astute she might identify different roles amongst the professionals, the largest groups of which she might call 'doctors', 'nurses', 'managers' and 'administrators'. Others ('patients') would come less frequently and often irregularly, usually for short periods but sometimes in those establishments she called 'hospitals' staying for days or even weeks, but never with the regular pattern of the professionals.

As MacIntyre reminds us institutions must not be confused with practices.[27] Yet it is perhaps reasonable on the basis of the description above to suggest that what goes on in the institutions we call hospitals and health centres are not separate practices of medicine, nursing, health service management, etc., but one common practice of health care. This is a socially established cooperative activity in which both health professionals and patients play particular roles, cultivate peculiar virtues and achieve their own internal goods, which contribute to the wellbeing of both.

Health care is not the only practice that includes different and asymmetrical roles. Team games involve players with different roles, each with their particular excellences: goalkeeper, beater, striker, seeker. Our imaginary Martian anthropologist might note that for many people being a football supporter or a cricket fan is an integral part of their narrative (including the opportunity to develop the virtue of fortitude when their team plays badly?). Similarly music and the theatre have a core of people who maintain the practice and to whose lives it is central, and a larger group who gain from it but for whom it is just one small element in their narrative.

But this is not passive consumption; any actor will tell you that a good or a bad audience makes a huge difference to the internal goods generated by a play. And although being an audience is an occasional activity, it still involves being inducted into the standards of excellence of the practice. One has to learn to hiss Ebenezer in *Aladdin* but not Iago in *Othello*; to shout 'he's behind you' to Buttons in *Cinderella* but not to Hamlet on the battlements of Elsinore. So perhaps it is reasonable to consider health care as a practice in the MacIntyrean sense: a complex and coherent socially organised activity in which patients, doctors, nurses, other clinicians, managers and administrators all play their roles, each making his particular contribution to achieving the standards of excellence characteristic of this practice and through that contribution obtaining the internal goods appropriate to his role.

If health care is a practice in MacIntyre's sense then it follows that through this cooperative activity human powers to achieve excellence are extended for all those engaged in it, whatever role they play. How this occurs will however differ for the two main groups who take part in the practice. For professionals the internal goods are similar to those which MacIntyre refers to in relation to both self-contained and purposive practices. They include the satisfaction of exercising analytic skill and strategic imagination, whether in making a diagnosis, carrying out an operation, designing a strategic plan for a hospital service or administering an appointment system efficiently. These resemble the internal goods of chess, one of MacIntyre's examples of a practice. They also involve more person-centred attributes – the development of relationships, the exercise of patience and the communication of feelings that resemble the internal goods of other practices as diverse as theatre and parenting. We will explore the internal goods that doctors obtain from their participation in the practice of health care and the virtues which contribute to those goods in more detail in Chapter 5.

For patients the internal goods are different. Aristotle[28] suggests that the good of medicine is health, and this is the principal internal good that, as patients, we seek through the practice of health care. How health care contributes to health and its place in the overall story of a life will be the subject of the next chapter.

For professionals and patients alike seeing health care as a practice may provide the moral coherence that is 'a partial solution'[29] to the fragmented discourse considered in the last chapter. Applying MacIntyre's concept of a practice to health care suggests that, rather than the conflicting goals of maximisation of quality-adjusted life years (QALYs) and health gain, efficient management to minimise costs, prolonging life and avoiding death, doing one's duty, following rules and avoiding legal challenge and providing patient satisfaction, the construction of better narratives for patients and professionals alike should be the focus of health care.

This view of health care as a collaborative practice involving both patients and professionals has implications for how professionals and patients relate to each other. It casts professionals and patients as collaborators in a struggle against suffering and incapacity: as 'co-producers of health'[30] rather than opponents. At first sight this seems similar to contemporary notions of partnership between clinicians and patients and patient-centred practice,[31] but conceiving this within a virtue ethic rather than in terms of an adversarial right or legalistic concept of patient autonomy or a consumerist view of patient satisfaction will affect the nature of the partnership. For both patients and practitioners a collaborative approach may be more productive of their respective internal goods than the expectation of conflict, or at best armed truce, which comes from the adversarial assumptions of deontological, legalist or consumerist models. In fact this may be closer to the experience many practitioners and patients already have. In spite of outside pressures encouraging patients to claim their rights and doctors to defend themselves from attack, clinicians and patients seem to get along pretty well with working together to address the patient's health problems most of the time.[32]

This understanding of health care may also offer a way out of the conflict between autonomy and beneficence that has dogged bioethics for a generation.[33] From the deontological perspective doctors have two, potentially conflicting, duties – to do the best for the patient and to respect her autonomy (two of Beauchamp and Childress's four principles[34] – or three if non-maleficence is merely seen as the other side of the beneficence coin). When patients do not want to do what the doctor thinks is clearly best these duties conflict. If however autonomy is seen not as a static concept, a moral or legal 'right', a possession to be treasured and protected from others, but instead is seen as an internal good, a capacity to be developed as we face the challenges of life, part of the human power to achieve excellence, an aspect of the virtues and *eudaemonia*, then the practice of health care becomes one way in which autonomy can be enhanced for those who participate as patients. Most obviously it can be enhanced by removing or ameliorating the challenges to autonomy posed by illness through curative treatment. But also it can be enhanced by finding a way to live a flourishing life within the limits fixed by disability and illness that cannot be cured. Patient and professional are not working in opposition on this, because both partners are seeking the same ends, contributing their different expertise to reach a shared understanding of a way forward that includes enhanced autonomy.

A practice amongst practices

One of the criticisms MacIntyre makes of modernity is that it partitions life into a variety of segments, each with its own norms and modes of behaviour.[35] Work and leisure, private and public life, are made into distinct realms. But if we view human life as a narrative unity, practices do not exist in isolation; they intertwine and reinforce each other. The virtues of the mother and the virtues of the doctor have distinct characteristics but also have much in common.

Balance is central to virtue ethics. A good life involves participation in a balanced range of practices. This is not the same as 'work–life balance' (for from MacIntyre's perspective work is part of life, not something apart from it) but rather a complementarity between the variety of practices we participate in. For both professionals and patients health care is one of a number of such practices that contribute to their unique personal life narrative. They may combine the practice of health care with parenting, music and marriage or other long-term relationships. If they engage in these sincerely, with commitment and with an appropriate balance, this will be a good narrative. Excessive emphasis on the practice of health care however may lead to a life that is stunted. In patients we call this hypochondria; in professionals we call it workaholism.

Can this work in a multicultural society?

We live in a culturally diverse society whose members have very different views of the purpose of life and how one should live. Is it possible to practise health care (or indeed any practice that contributes to individual and social wellbeing) on a teleological basis in a society where people's goals and values are so varied, a society that includes agnostics, Christians, Muslims, Jews and militant atheists? MacIntyre seems certain that concepts such as virtue, justice and rationality only make sense within a tradition or a community.[36] Does this mean that a MacIntyrean approach to health care with its emphasis on tradition, social cooperation and the genesis of virtues and the internal goods cannot work in a pluralist society?

Moral relativism, the idea that in a pluralist society there is such a diversity of values and goals that it is impossible to make moral judgements, is widespread in our post-Enlightenment, post-modern society. It is often associated with emotivism, the view that values are non-rational matters of taste and '*de gustibus non est disputandum*'. Midgley[37] however argues convincingly that, although cultures vary, they share a common basis in our shared, biologically determined, human nature and the nature of the world in which we live. There is a lot more commonality in values between those with different religions and value systems than at first sight appears. She gives the example of different funeral customs: one culture buries its dead, another exposes them on towers for their flesh to be picked off by birds, another burns the bodies. Each may find the custom of the others abhorrent, but they are all expressions of one fundamental shared value – one should treat the dead bodies of one's loved ones with respect.

The sense that life has a purpose and a shape is perhaps a similar fundamental value. Whether or not they use such a term, most people in most cultures see *eudaemonia* as involving participation in family and personal relationships, work (paid or unpaid, within or outside the home), and growth as an individual through education and emotional and spiritual experiences. There may be differences of emphasis on the importance of these different elements of *eudaemonia* between different individuals and groups that need to be understood and acknowledged, but apart from those few, such as suicide bombers and others who wish to break down the fabric of society, the values we share across social groups are more fundamental than our differences.

Health care is likely to be particularly close to this shared inheritance because it is grounded in factors fundamental to human nature and experience: our common physiology and anatomy, our basic biological functions and our shared mortality. There will of course be issues on the margins where there are differences, but these should not blind us to the importance of these shared core values or take an overdue proportion of our ethical attention (as they are sometimes inclined to do).

Cultural and individual differences will of course affect what makes a good narrative for each of us. Aristotle points out[38] that the most desirable activity for an individual depends on his disposition. Since there are wide varieties of practices, each with its peculiar internal goods, our choice of practices will be determined by our disposition, which will depend on our innate gifts as well as our choices. But there will be some general principles (what Hursthouse calls 'v-rules'[39]) about how participation in health care contributes to this for both patients and professionals. The nature of these general principles in the life of patients is the subject of the next chapter.

Notes

1. Kuhn TS. *The Structure of Scientific Revolutions*. Chicago: University of Chicago Press, 1962.

2. MacIntyre A. *After Virtue: a study in moral theory* (2nd edn). London: Duckworth, 1985.

3. Pellegrino ED, Thomasma DC. *The Virtues in Medical Practice*. New York: Oxford University Press, 1993.

4. Pellegrino ED, Thomasma DC. *Christian Virtues in Medical Practice*. Washington, DC: Georgetown University Press, 1996.

5. Aristotle. *The Ethics of Aristotle: the Nicomachean ethics* (trans. JAK Thomson). Harmondsworth: Penguin, 1955.

6. Aquinas, St Thomas. *Summa Theologica* (Prima Secundæ Partis). Cambridge: Cambridge University Press, 1990; Latin original and English translation, www.newadvent.org/summa/2.htm [accessed 16 January 2014].

7. MacIntyre. *After Virtue*, p. 191.

8. MacIntyre. *After Virtue*, p. 187.

9. MacIntyre. *After Virtue*, p. 193.

10. MacIntyre. *After Virtue*, p. 193.

11. MacIntyre. *After Virtue*, p. 190.

12. MacIntyre. *After Virtue*, p. 190.

13. MacIntyre. *After Virtue*, p. 190.

14. MacIntyre. *After Virtue*, p. 194.

15. MacIntyre. *After Virtue*, p. 190.

16. MacIntyre. *After Virtue*, p. 190.

17. MacIntyre. *After Virtue*, p. 190.

18. MacIntyre. *After Virtue*, p. 188.

19. MacIntyre. *After Virtue*, p. 188

20. Miller D. Virtues, practices and justice. In: J Horton, S Mendus (eds), *After MacIntyre*. Cambridge: Cambridge University Press, 1994, pp. 245–64.

21. MacIntyre A. Patients as agents. In: SF Spicker, HT Engelhart (eds), *Philosophical Medical Ethics, Its Nature and Significance*. Dordrecht/Boston: D. Reidel Co., 1977, pp. 197–212, http://wfbinst.org/medicine.pdf [accessed 1 May 2014].

22. Hippocrates. Aphorisms, § 1.1. http://classics.mit.edu/Hippocrates/aphorisms.1.i.html [accessed 16 January 2014].

23. Tyson P. The Hippocratic oath today. 2001. www.pbs.org/wgbh/nova/body/hippocratic-oath-today.html [accessed 16 January 2014].

24. Department of Health. Modernisation of health and care. News, information and conversations. http://webarchive.nationalarchives.gov.uk/20130805112926/http://healthandcare.dh.gov.uk [accessed 16 January 2014].

25. General Medical Council. *Leadership and Management for All Doctors*. London: GMC, p. 20, www.gmc-uk.org/static/documents/content/LM_guidance.pdf [accessed 16 January 2014].

26. Cameron D. I see managerialism as a virus. *Guardian*, 4 April 2002, www.guardian.co.uk/society/2002/apr/05/publicvoices4 [accessed 16 January 2014].

27. MacIntyre. *After Virtue*, p. 194.

28. Aristotle. *The Ethics of Aristotle*, Book I, p. 63.

29. MacIntyre. *After Virtue*, p. 201.

30. Hart JT. *A New Kind of Doctor*. London: Merlin Press, 1988.

31. International Alliance of Patients' Organizations. *What is Patient-Centred Health Care? A review of definitions and principles*. London: IAPO, 2007, www.patientsorganizations.org/pchreview [accessed 16 January 2014].

32. Patient satisfaction with GP services is high, survey shows. *BMJ Careers*, 24 July 2008, http://careers.bmj.com/careers/advice/view-article.html?id=3023 [accessed 16 January 2014].

33. O'Neill O. *Autonomy and Trust in Bioethics* (the Gifford Lectures 2001). Cambridge: Cambridge University Press, 2002, http://catdir.loc.gov/catdir/samples/cam033/2002073521.pdf [accessed 16 January 2014].

34. Beauchamp TL, Childress JF. *Principles of Biomedical Ethics*. New York: Oxford University Press, 1989.

35. MacIntyre. *After Virtue*, Chapter 15, p. 204.

36. MacIntyre A. *Three Rival Versions of Moral Enquiry*. London: Duckworth, 1990.

37. Midgley M. *Can't We Make Moral Judgements?* Bristol: Bristol Press, 1991.

38. Aristotle. *Ethics*, Book X.

39. Hursthouse R. *Applying Virtue Ethics: study guide* (Open University course A432). Buckingham: Open University, 2000, Part II § 6.

Chapter 3

Flourishing and the internal goods of the practice

When Aristotle said that the good of medicine is health[1] he was giving an illustration to explain what he meant by the good at which an activity aims. He did not discuss in any detail the nature of the good of health, its contribution to the cultivation of the virtues and the development of a flourishing narrative, or the place of health care within this scheme. Nor does MacIntyre have very much to say on this. The purpose of this chapter is to try to build on their more general thinking to explore these issues.

As I suggested in Chapter 1, we must distinguish clearly between health and health care. In Miller's terminology[2] health is the purpose of the practice of health care; it is the principal internal good that comes from participation in the practice for patients. Health care exists to promote good health in the same way as architecture exists to produce good buildings, and both are essential parts of the infrastructure of a good life. Therefore to understand the nature of a flourishing practice of health care, we need a vision of what a good life is, and how health contributes to such a life.

What is *eudaemonia*?

Aristotle's *Ethics* is an exploration of what sort of life we should seek to live (or possibly notes for a series of lectures on the subject). The word Aristotle uses for this is *eudaemonia*, which is often translated as 'a good life'. The problem with this rendering is that, like many widely used terms in English (virtue, charity), it can carry implicit values that are not necessarily those we would consciously espouse.[3] Saying someone has led a good life may be thought to mean that they have spent their life doing good things for others (or at least refrained from obvious harm) with Kantian undertones, whilst living the good life might suggest a life of pleasure, with hedonistic implications (unless one has in mind the 1970s sit-com *The Good Life*,[4] which portrayed a third vision: a life of simplicity, self-sufficiency and rejection of materialism – Jean-Jacques Rousseau[5] meets St Francis of Assisi[6]). Another common translation of *eudaemonia* is happiness. Again this is a slippery word with various meanings – pleasure, contentment or fulfilment, or a combination of all three; it needs clarification if we are to use it to define the purpose of our lives.

In Book I of the *Ethics* Aristotle summarily dismisses the view that *eudaemonia* is a life that seeks to maximise pleasure as a bovine view of the servile masses.[7] In Book X he offers a more nuanced discussion[8] in which he concludes that though pleasure is A good, it does not make sense to see it as THE Good, because we seek more from life than pleasure. This seems to fit with what we can infer about most people's values from their lives. Although they enjoy pleasure, people give it up and undergo hardship, discomfort and even danger to achieve goals such as giving their children a good education, conquering Everest, or working to make the world a better place as they see it. This suggests that, for most people, although pleasure may be welcomed it is not the fundamental goal of their lives.

Contentment as the essence of the good life is similarly limited. There is much to be said for acceptance of what has to be rather than perpetually striving for the unattainable (which is a problem for consequentialism, since maximum good is by definition always out of reach), but contentment can be only a little less bovine than pleasure. A cow chewing the cud in a field of lush grass on a fine day seems to be the acme of contentment, but as an image for the purpose of human life it seems to lack something, as Huxley made clear in *Brave New World*.[9] It is too static an idea to be more than a partial element of *eudaemonia*.

Happiness as fulfilment is perhaps a more satisfactory understanding of *eudaemonia*, because it implies that life has a purpose (*telos*) – Maslow's self-actualisation. But it doesn't give us much guidance on how we decide whether someone is fulfilled or not, and like contentment it is somewhat static – once you are fulfilled, what then?

Another translation sometimes used for *eudaemonia* is flourishing, and I'm inclined to think that this is perhaps the best English term. It is a dynamic, botanical metaphor, which incorporates the idea of fulfilment of a purpose but also the shape and narrative of a lifelong process. The word comes from the Latin *florere*, to blossom or flower. Its more general use to mean succeeding or thriving in body, mind or spirit is a metaphorical extension of this literal botanical meaning. In our youth-obsessed and death-averse culture it is easy to think of flourishing and health solely in terms of the early stages of life when powers are growing and fruit is borne, but a cycle of germination, growth, flowering, the production of spores, seed or fruit followed by decay and death is common to all plant life. A flourishing plant will go through all these stages in due season, and each has its place. At the appropriate time seedpods and dead-heads are as much evidence of flourishing as buds and flowers, and may be as beautiful a part of the garden and as essential to a successful life cycle as a plant in full bloom.

This metaphor implies that for life to be worthwhile it has to have both shape and meaning. It is a flourishing *narrative*, a story with a beginning and middle and end, and like any good story it has a meaning. Life is not just one damned thing after another, the game of Consequences discussed in Chapter 1, a tale told by an idiot, sound and fury signifying nothing.[10] This does not mean that setbacks may not be part of that narrative; pruning in the short term may seem painful and even disastrous, but may ultimately lead to greater flourishing and a life of greater beauty.

This understanding of the nature of life implies an acceptance of death as part of life, which has important implications for health care. Heath[11] recently argued that current approaches to treatment (essentially consequentialist), which seek to postpone death at all costs, ignore the fact that death is inevitable, and must have some cause and some nature. Despite the popularity of the phrase in headlines, slick quotes and advertising slogans,[12] lives are never saved; deaths are merely postponed. And if we see life as a narrative with a purpose, postponing death does not always make a life better. A good death as well as a good life is important, even if the cost of a good death is a shorter life. A commitment to flourishing may mean rejecting possible but probably futile medical interventions.

A friend of mine died recently at the age of 93. When she was 90 she was diagnosed with bowel cancer. She had lived and continued to live a flourishing life. Although she was still active her sight and hearing were failing. She had diabetes, was unsteady on her feet and suffered with osteoporotic back pain. She resisted considerable pressure to undergo surgery and chemotherapy for her tumour in the belief that the suffering and disability these treatments would involve was not worthwhile, and she would have a better life and a better death without them.

Whether she was right or not we cannot tell, but given that the average life expectancy of a woman at 90 (many of whom presumably will not have been diagnosed with a terminal illness) is little more than four years,[13] it was not an unreasonable view. What actually happened was that she lived a full and active life for more than two years after making that decision, until a fall started the downward spiral that ended in her peaceful death nine months later.

In contrast to this story, many clinicians will have seen patients spend their last days in a futile fight against death, often encouraged to do so by healthcare professionals and/or relatives who see death as the ultimate failure. Making the choice not to do this in a culture where fear of death and a consequentialist understanding of the good life are common demands considerable determination and courage. My friend's courage in the face of death was demonstrated a few months before she died when, over a convivial dinner, she invited me to her funeral. At that funeral, at her request, after a moving Requiem Mass her body was carried out to the triumphant final movement of the Saint-Saëns Organ Symphony.[14]

The illustration on the cover of the General Medical Council (GMC) end-of-life guidance[15] is of autumn leaves: an acknowledgement of the botanical metaphor of flourishing that both illustrates the inevitability of decay and death, but also recognises that it is not entirely negative – autumn leaves are one of the most beautiful aspects of nature.

Aristotle's view of how to achieve a flourishing life

Aristotle concluded that the two most important elements in a flourishing life are friendship[16] and contemplation.[17] Again we need to be careful that we don't make mistakes about what he meant because of unexamined assumptions about the words we use to translate him. We tend to use the word contemplation to mean silent gazing, perhaps in the context of monasticism or some other religious or meditative activity: ways of life that did not exist in Aristotle's lifetime. Both from his discussion and from his life, it would seem that Aristotle's idea of contemplation was far wider than this. He studied and wrote books on nature as well as on sociology, philosophy and ethics;[18] so perhaps for Aristotle contemplation included understanding, classification and analysis as well as the wordless wonderment the word immediately suggests to us. When considering *eudaemonia* it might make more sense to think in terms of this broader vision of contemplation.

Our idea of friendship will also be different from that of Aristotle. He was writing for a rather narrow audience – male, educated and leisured, a world from which women, slaves and even probably free men who were uneducated and lived by manual labour were excluded. The idea of genuine friendship between men and women, as part of sexual and family relationships, and between colleagues and those we meet in our work, would have been foreign to him. Here perhaps our broader vision is more useful than Aristotle's.

So although we can use Aristotle's idea that friendship and contemplation lie at the heart of *eudaemonia* to help us explore the role of health care in promoting flourishing, these terms may mean something very different for us because we live in a different world. Ethics, like other practices, has grown and developed in the 2000 years since Aristotle wrote, as our understanding of the nature of the world and of human nature has grown through many academic disciplines and other human activities. This means that we may have a richer idea of the goods of understanding and of relationships than were available to him, although we should be careful not to be too sure that this is the case. Whitehead famously described European philosophy (including Aristotle) as merely a set of footnotes to Plato,[19] and to borrow the well-known image used by Sir Isaac Newton,[20] even if we can see further than either of those giants, we can only do so because we are standing on their shoulders.

Health and the flourishing life

Doyal and Gough have argued convincingly[21] that good health is a core human need, a prerequisite for flourishing in many other ways. It is also however itself part of what it means to flourish, just as virtue is both necessary for flourishing and part of a flourishing life. But this cannot mean health in the original World Health Organization (WHO) definition as a complete state of physical and mental wellbeing.[22] Such a concept of health for all is unrealistic, because it ignores the reality of illness, disability and death as part of every life, sometimes avoidable but not always or for ever. Such a broad definition also tends to medicalise problems (particularly psychological ones) that are not necessarily best thought of in terms of health and illness.

A more recent WHO definition of mental health as 'a state of well-being in which every individual realizes his or her own potential, can cope with the normal stresses of life, can work productively and fruitfully, and is able to make a contribution to her or his community' is perhaps more realistic for both physical and mental health.[23] It is close to Huber's notion of health[24] as the ability to adapt and to self-manage. His biologically rooted concept of allostasis is very close to the concept of flourishing discussed above, but it does not address how we deal with situations where allostasis breaks down and cannot be fully restored. This is when potential, coping and contribution to society are limited by health problems that cannot be prevented or overcome by biomedical intervention: disability, disabling acute illness and chronic disease. And of course, although we may shrink from accepting this, death is sooner or later inevitable for all of us. We need an understanding of health that enables us to flourish despite these limitations. What additional insights does seeing health care as a MacIntyrean practice in the Aristotelian tradition give us?

The contribution of biomedical health care to flourishing

In *What is Good General Practice?*[25] I argued that health care promoted three different types of good. The most obvious is action to relieve suffering and cure disease using the powerful biomedical model. The contribution this makes to flourishing is fairly obvious: pain and incapacity limit our ability to engage in other practices that contribute to a flourishing narrative. One of the undoubted triumphs of health care is its ability – through antibiotics, surgery, chemotherapy and similar interventions – to prevent flourishing lives being brought to a premature end. 'Cut down in their prime' is a phrase that extends the botanical metaphor. In the 1970s Julian Tudor Hart[26] and others criticised this as mopping up the floor without turning off the taps, and since then the emphasis on the use of the powerful biomedical model to prevent rather than cure disease has grown enormously, particularly in general practice. The ability of computerised records to allow us to measure what we have not done has made it possible to move prevention to the centre of health care.

As is often the case society is one step behind science in this respect, and most patients still come to their doctors expecting treatment for existing problems rather than for problems they do not yet have, which can produce tensions in the consultation that make many doctors uncomfortable.[27] The clinician is encouraged by the Quality and Outcomes Framework (QOF) and the electronic reminders it has spawned to check blood pressure and record smoking and alcohol consumption, whilst patients want something to make their sore throats go away. The tension between meeting the need the patient presents and addressing the risk factors for those he does not yet have can also pose problems for the clinician.[28]

Prevention, alleviation and cure can of course contribute to flourishing. Some preventive activities have a minimal effect on life narrative, but offer considerable benefit; hand washing and immunisation are obvious examples. Others enhance autonomy and the richness of life; exercise for weight loss and muscle strengthening for back pain are examples of preventive activities that have benefits beyond the biomedical, and which are likely to enhance flourishing. Others move patients from the kingdom of the well to the kingdom of the sick[29] for benefits that are less clear. Screening for prostate cancer, with its uncertain meaning and risk of increasing anxiety,[30] is one example of such an intervention. Heath suggested that screening for depression in patients with diabetes might be another, tantamount to saying 'you've got one chronic disease; would you like another?'[31]

Conditions that are risk factors for disease (hypertension, hypercholester-olaemia) are often seen as illnesses in themselves, which can make people see themselves as ill and increase anxiety or guilt. If the purpose of health care is to promote flourishing narratives perhaps we need to evaluate preventive activities in that context, encouraging those that contribute to flourishing, and being wary of those likely to impair it.

It also implies being more careful about the language we use when discussing risk factors and screening tests, talking perhaps of 'extending lives' rather than saving them, and being careful to distinguish between risk factors and illnesses. Perhaps too we need to be more cautious in making judgements about the value of screening tests and preventive interventions. We can make general judgements about the value of these, but ultimately the decision will depend on the patient and her individual life narrative. One patient may benefit from the reduction in cardiovascular risk from taking antihypertensive or cholesterol-lowering drugs without any adverse effects or worrying about their implication; another may suffer disabling muscle aches or dizziness, or have his self-confidence or sense of wellbeing gravely harmed by a diagnosis of hypertension or hypercholester-olaemia.

Managerialism and legalism tend to discourage professionals from *phronesis* when advising patients on decisions like this. QOF targets are based on absolute rates of activity, irrespective of individual circumstances, and although there are arrangements for 'exception reporting' clinicians may feel under pressure to include as many patients as possible. Or clinicians feel constrained to ensure that their practice is 'NICE compliant' (sometimes by external managerialist pressure, but perhaps as often by their own 'inner managerialist') and worry they may be medico-legally vulnerable if they don't follow guidelines. Clinicians experience these fears despite two successive chairmen of the National Institute for Health and Care Excellence (NICE)[32,33] having stated publicly (in my hearing) that guidelines are guidance, and that they would expect that sometimes there will be good reasons (particularly patient choice or co-morbidity) for not following them. Evidence-based medicine is sometimes unfairly blamed for this situation, but it is more likely to be another result of the internalisation of the values of legalism and managerialism discussed in Chapter 1. The 'father' of evidence-based medicine Dr David Sackett was clear that evidence-based practice meant using the best available research evidence *combined with professional judgement and patient values*,[34] but this aspect of his definition is commonly overlooked.

The contribution of interpretative health care to flourishing

Many people go to their GP not principally because they want to change what is happening to them but because they want to understand it. Is it serious or trivial? Will it get better, and how quickly? What impact will it have on their work, their family life, their social and sporting activities? Answering questions like these is an important aspect of health care, for which clinicians are often ill-equipped by their basic education. It is part of the third aspect of health care, the interpretative function – giving prognostic information and helping patients understand their illness.

At one time doctors could make diagnoses and give prognoses, but their therapeutic interventions were of limited value (indeed often counter-productive). The interpretative function was then a large part of what they had to offer. The development of scientific medicine as part of the Enlightenment project has made diagnosis and prognosis more accurate, but it has also increased the range of effective therapeutic interventions enormously. As a result treatment has come to be seen as the main activity of health care – and thus the randomised controlled trial, the most rigorous way to assess the impact of an intervention, is seen as the gold standard of medical knowledge.

But if the main purpose of medicine is to help patients construct a flourishing narrative, then it follows that the interpretative function should be at the heart of practice. Properly used it empowers patients to deal with illness appropriately, so they can overcome it when that is possible and 'bear what must be borne'[35] when it is not.

This does not of course mean ignoring biomedical intervention. Often such treatment is an important part of creating a new and better narrative for the patient. But if the purpose of health care is to help patients to construct a flourishing narrative, biomedical treatment and biomedical prevention are secondary to the interpretative function, because how we interpret what is happening is more important than what is actually happening. This is the opposite of the usual prioritisation that sees biomedical treatment as the main purpose of medicine, biomedical prevention second and the interpretative function as an almost optional extra.

Within a MacIntyrean framework the interpretative function is not just about explanation of pathophysiology and prognosis, although these are important. Understanding our bodies is not just a source of intellectual curiosity and wonder (though it can be both); it is part of understanding what it is to be human in general, and more specifically to be the person we are, with our own particular frailties and capacities. In a climate of post-Enlightenment dualism it is easy to see our 'selves' as purely mental constructs, and our bodies as packaging, no more part of 'us' than a hotel room in which we sleep and eat for a while is a home. But human beings are better thought of as embodied minds, and understanding the capacities and limitations of our bodies is an aspect of *phronesis* – as important to flourishing as an understanding of our emotional responses and intellectual powers. Health care can help us do this, and in a way it is part of contemplation, one of Aristotle's ends of the flourishing life.

But health care is not only concerned with understanding our bodies and our minds in the way history is concerned with understanding the past or astronomy with understanding the universe. The purpose of health care is to apply that understanding to produce the purposive good of health care, health, for patients. Participation in the interpretative function of health care with clinicians can be one way in which people construct that aspect of their narrative that deals with health and illness, life and death. Once the patient has an understanding of what is happening, she must decide how to respond to it. She may see herself as a hero, a victim or a helper;[36] she may have an internal or an external 'locus of control';[37] her story may be one of supplication, deliverance or self-sacrifice.[38] The role of the clinician is to help patients construct the best possible narrative – to write a life story that helps them maximise their virtues and flourish, which fulfils their potential and sets them free.

To help patients create flourishing narratives interpretation has to make development and growth possible; it has to be a narrative of empowerment as well as of understanding. Not all interpretation does this. For example, I have seen patients for whom psychotherapy has provided interpretations that give them enormous understanding of their situation and its causes but which still leave them powerless to change anything for the better. They can give a very clear account of their poor self-image, its roots in their childhood experiences and how this leads to anxiety, poor social functioning and impoverished relationships, but they have no tools that enable them to use this understanding to improve their lives. Understanding one's psychic functioning can make a significant contribution to development and flourishing, but without learning how to use that understanding to improve their story then its contribution is severely limited. Indeed, if it makes someone see themselves as powerless victims of circumstances it may have the opposite effect; they may see their personality disorder or their obsessive-compulsive disorder (OCD) as part of their fate beyond their control. This implies that cognitive-behavioural therapy, where therapists and patients work on how to make changes as well as why things happen, may often be preferable to some analytic approaches which assume that change will follow understanding.

Health care and the goods of relationships

Making sense of how to live with illness, disability and death, and flourish within their unavoidable limitations, is the only 'healthy' way in which health care can contribute to flourishing and virtue. To understand how it can do this we need to consider how the interpretative function of health care works.

The relationship between clinician and patient is crucial. Health care does not primarily exist to bring people together; it exists to understand and cope with illness, and in one way or another to overcome it. But this internal good is the product of a relationship between patient and clinician that can perhaps be partly understood in terms of friendship.

Aristotle devotes two books of the *Ethics* to consideration of friendship,[39] which he makes clear he sees as an important element in the flourishing life. But in the male-dominated Greek *polis*, where social relationships, study, politics and sex were combined in ways that would seem strange to us, friendship meant something very different from what it does today. Aristotle was a product of his time – he accepted slavery and the subjugation of women without question[40] – and I suspect if we were to meet him today we would think he was something of a snob. Two thousand years of Christian emphasis on the importance of brotherly love since his time has produced not only the cuckoo clock[41] but also an awareness of the value of relationships with people from a wide variety of backgrounds. In contrast to Ancient Greece, for most of us friendship might include our life partners, our family and others with whom we share our domestic life: all relationships that produce internal goods. And we might want to include in our definition of the goods of relationship all of Lewis's four loves,[42] *eros, storge, agape* – erotic love, familial affection, and the love of humanity – as well as *philos*, the love shown in friendship.

Aristotle was fairly dismissive of utilitarian relationships,[43] and perhaps compared with selfless friendships in which people enjoy each other's company for its own sake, which he considers the highest form of friendship, he was right. But the relationships we make at work with colleagues and the much more casual relationships with those we share our leisure activities – fellow choristers, people in our night-school class, and even the casual contacts of daily life, such as the newsagent, the lady in the bread shop, the postman, the builder – can also enrich our lives. In the same way, when the practice of health care is flourishing it includes a wide variety of relationships that contribute to flourishing for those involved: relationships between professionals and patients for both parties, and for professionals relationships with other professionals of disparate types.

As patients the relationships we make through our engagement in the practice of health care are most of the time on a par with the utilitarian relationships mentioned above, particularly when the emphasis is on the biomedical and preventive functions. Having a good doctor or nurse is akin to having a good plumber or cleaner, or a nice lady in the shop on the corner who sells you good bread whilst exchanging a cheery word: a necessary part of the infrastructure of life, which if it works well adds a little joy and richness beyond the merely utilitarian exchange, but not at the heart of life.

This is what we should expect to be a patient's experience of health care in a flourishing practice with problems that can easily be solved; they should see their doctors, nurses and receptionists as helpful friends rather than as servants from whom they demand services as of right, authority figures who control access to services they need, or vendors whose goods they acquire through payment. But for some of us, at key points in our lives when we have problems that have to be lived with rather than solved, these relationships mean far more than that. The relationship with the doctor when it goes well can be a healing one ('the drug doctor').[44] It may well be part of the means by which the placebo effect works.[45] It is often the relationship between clinician and patient that makes the interpretative function effective in promoting flourishing.[46] Illness narratives are produced in a performance in which both doctor and patient take part. The virtuous practitioner is someone who helps people produce good narratives, but she needs the support of a virtuous patient too (or rather both doctor and practitioner need to aspire to virtue). It takes two to tango.

How to dance the interpretative tango

An aspect of medical practice frequently overlooked is that of accompanying the patient on the journey of illness. Heath speaks of the doctor as witness;[47] a helpful concept, although the doctor's role is rarely that of a passive bystander in the way we usually think of witnesses in court cases. It is more akin to a companion or guide through the dark wood[48] of illness (and the even darker wood of the health service!). Perhaps a related, more active sense of witness is helpful here, that used when people talk of witness in relation to religious faith. In this specialised use of the term witnessing is not just watching passively, but speaking out and acting in accordance with a belief in what has been seen and experienced. The Greek word in the New Testament usually translated as witness is *martyria*, and martyrs are so called because their death for what they believed to be the truth was the ultimate witness in this sense. Medical witnesses are fortunately rarely required to undergo martyrdom, but perhaps the role of the GP as a witness is rather more active than just writing it down, as the 'clerk of the community'.[49] It involves bringing together the general facts of medical science with the particular facts that the patient shares with the doctor, and working with the patient to produce a more hopeful and hence more flourishing narrative. And like martyrdom this sometimes requires courage as well as vision, although this undramatic variety of moral courage is perhaps better referred to as fortitude.

In a famous portrait from the pre-antibiotic era the doctor is just holding the patient's hand, gazing into space; in those days pretty much all one could do as one waited and prayed that the natural strength of the body would enable the patient to survive the crisis and the fever to abate. He isn't doing anything – he is just there. Paul Julian talks of the importance of the doctor 'being there'[50] in modern general practice, but perhaps because there is so much more we can do these days, the importance of the doctor just 'being there' is easily overlooked. This is odd, because amongst younger people 'he's always there for me' has become a common way of expressing the value of a relationship.

Figure 3.1: Lawrence Alma-Tadema's *Portrait of Dr Washington Epps, My Doctor*[51]

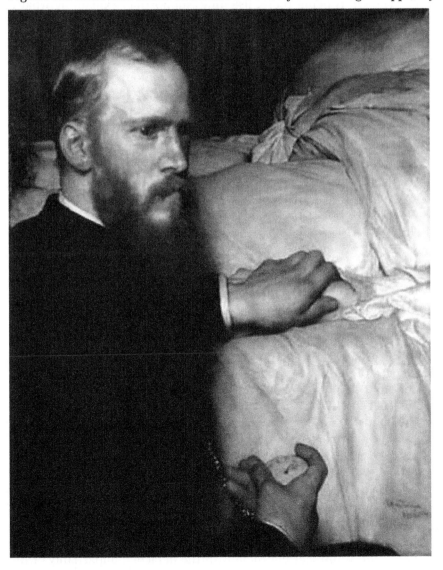

'Being there' can be important in many situations:[52]

- A patient has a worrying symptom: a breast lump, an area of numbness, some swollen glands, dysphagia. The GP identifies the problem, explains the reason for her concern and agrees with the patient a referral process, these days in the UK usually under the two-week wait process. In practical terms her job is done – it is now up to the specialist to make the assessment, organise relevant investigations, make a diagnosis and advise on treatment. Sometimes referral is the limit of GP involvement, but sometimes at the initiative of doctor or patient further consultations take place, alongside hospital investigations and treatments. The GP is being there, listening, supporting, explaining what is going on; this can be invaluable but takes fortitude.

- A parent brings a toddler in, with symptoms of a viral infection. The illness itself is obviously trivial, but the parental anxiety arises from past history: the child has previously had a febrile convulsion, or pneumonia in the first year of life, or has some congenital anomaly. Nothing can be done to alter the course of events. The doctor's job is just to be there, encouraging and comforting (in the original sense of *con forte* – with strength).

- A patient is terminally ill at home, and the doctor visits for symptom control or to assess a new problem. The patient's partner offers a cup of tea, and it feels right to accept it (though it is not actually wanted, and has far too much milk). The tea is accepted because the doctor's job is to be there. The conversation over the tea may be trivial, or it may be the thing the doctor does that day that makes the most difference.

What does 'being there' mean in these and similar cases? It is slightly different from the 'being there for me' of friendship – being a shoulder to cry on, someone to offer an encouraging word, though it may include these, albeit in a rather more detached 'professional' way. In a way when 'being there' the doctor is acting more like a friend than as a professional, but it is a particular sort of friendship that is rooted in professional expertise and with professional boundaries. So, for example, part of the encouragement might come from the professional knowledge that most children who have pneumonia don't get it again, though they continue to get colds: from an understanding of what an endoscopy involves, which when explained in a familiar environment can be more easily taken in than during a hospital visit. The support offered may include a pat on the arm and a kind word, but it is unlikely to include the hug or the suggestion of a visit to the pub that a friend might offer as part of 'being there'.

The term 'reassurance' is traditionally used in medical circles in situations like these. This concept is viewed with scepticism within the Balint movement because it often means merely telling the patient there is no cause for concern. This has little impact unless the doctor understands the patient's concerns, enters into them with 'one head' whilst viewing them with the detached impartiality of the other head,[53] and then discusses both why the concern is understandable and why it is perhaps disproportionate or ill-founded, in language that makes sense to the patient. If this can be done then the patient goes away genuinely reassured. En-couraged is perhaps a better term, because the conversation has provided a 'transfusion' of the transmissible virtue of courage that helps the patient face realistic fears and casts out those with no foundation in reality.

The relation between health, health care, other practices and flourishing narratives

One of MacIntyre's criticisms of modernity is that it partitions life into segments, each with its own norms and modes of behaviour.[54] Work and leisure, private and public life, are seen as distinct, unconnected realms. But if human life is a narrative unity practices do not exist in isolation. For both professionals and patients health care is just one of a number of practices they engage in that contribute to their unique personal life narrative. So they may combine the practice of health care with parenting, music, marriage and other long-term relationships. If they engage in these practices sincerely and with commitment they intertwine and reinforce each other. The virtues of the mother, the doctor, the singer, the wife and the friend have distinct characteristics, but they have much in common. Successful participation in one practice contributes to success in another, and a narrative of flourishing will result.

Aristotle's idea that a virtue lies in a mean between two vices is not always true, and is little help in defining the virtues, but balance is important in the virtuous life.[55] It is characteristic of a flourishing narrative that there is a balance between the range of practices which make up that life. The right balance is not necessarily the same for each one of us and may change over time. Aristotle points out[56] that the most desirable activity for an individual depends on his disposition, and goes on to say that therefore to the good man virtuous activity is most desirable. Since however there are wide varieties of practices in which we can engage virtuously, our choice of practices will also be determined by our disposition, which in turn depends on our innate gifts as well as our choices.

We will say more about how the practice of health care contributes to flourishing for professionals in Chapter 5. For patients for much of the time health care is akin to sanitary engineering; it is part of the underpinning of a flourishing life, and like sanitary engineering should be unobtrusive and best hidden. But when we face those challenges in life best understood in terms of health it moves, at least for a while, to centre stage.

Challenges contribute to the cultivation of the virtues

Nussbaum and Sen[57] suggest that the virtues are the qualities we need to overcome the challenges of our life. Illness is a challenge we all face, sooner or later, and like other challenges it provides a training ground for developing virtues. The virtues we develop on these training grounds are transferable. The virtues we need to cope with a cold, commuting on the tube, and the traumas of buying a house are similar – courage, patience, respect for other people, etc. Success in overcoming these minor challenges helps us prepare for the major challenges of bereavement, life-threatening illness and death, the final and greatest challenge of all.

We see glimmerings of this tradition amongst patients. Some are reluctant to take medication not because they deny the abnormality or the unpleasantness of their experience or doubt that the medicine will work, but because they don't want to 'give in' to illness, to admit the weakness that accepting external assistance and the passivity of a patient implies They want to own their illness and overcome it. Metaphors of battle (I want to fight it, I don't want to give in) are commonly used; they want to see themselves as heroes, not victims. In an illness that is a challenge which can be overcome this can lead to a good narrative. Even when faced with an insurmountable challenge this may be an indication of courage in the face of adversity, but at other times it is a foolhardy rejection of practical help and an unwillingness to accept the reality of human frailty. Heroism isn't always possible, particularly near the end of life. Obituaries often speak of a long fight against a terminal illness, but this is a battle doomed to failure, tragic rather than heroic.

A flourishing life has various stages: development, maturity and the bearing of fruit, finally decay ending in death. All stages provide opportunities for cultivation of the virtues, and hence flourishing, albeit in different ways. In facing any challenge we need to ask four questions:

- What are the problems?

- What can we do to change them?

- What can't we do anything to change?

- How can we live with that and flourish despite it?

In health care the first three questions are the province of biomedicine, whilst the last requires the virtues developed through the interpretative function. The practicalities of working this out in any particular situation depend to a considerable extent on our definition of illnesses and our views of appropriate treatments, which we will consider in the next chapter.

Notes

1. Aristotle. *The Ethics of Aristotle: the Nicomachean ethics* (trans. JAK Thomson). Harmondsworth: Penguin, 1955, Book I § i.

2. Miller D. Virtues, practices and justice. In: J Horton, S Mendus (eds), *After MacIntyre.* Cambridge: Polity Press, 1994.

3. Toon PD. *Towards a Philosophy of General Practice* (Occasional Paper 78). London: RCGP, 1998.

4. *The Good Life.* BBC Comedy, www.bbc.co.uk/comedy/goodlife [accessed 16 January 2014].

5. Noble savage. *Encyclopaedia Britannica,* www.britannica.com/EBchecked/topic/416988/noble-savage [accessed 16 January 2014].

6. The Uncloistered Mystic. St Francis and holy poverty. 2001. http://theuncloisteredmystic.wordpress.com/2011/08/05/st-francis-and-holy-poverty [accessed 16 January 2014].

7. Aristotle. *Ethics,* Book I § v 1095b14.

8. Aristotle. *Ethics,* Book X § i–iv.

9. Huxley A. *Brave New World.* 1932. www.huxley.net/bnw.

10. Shakespeare W. *The Tragedy of Macbeth,* Act 5, Scene 5, http://shakespeare.mit.edu/macbeth/macbeth.5.5.html [accessed 16 January 2014].

11. Heath I. *Matters of Life and Death.* Abingdon: Radcliffe Publishing, 2007.

12. Some examples can be found by a search on 'save lives' at the quotation database Search Quotes, www.searchquotes.com/search/Save_Lives [accessed 16 January 2014].

13. The life expectancy tables at AnnuityAdvantage.com (www.annuityadvantage.com/lifeexpectancy.htm) give 4.6 years [accessed 16 January 2014]. The life expectancy calculator provided by Invidion financial calculators (www.invidion.co.uk/countdown_to_death.php) produces a result of 4.25 years [accessed 16 January 2014].

14. Saint-Saëns C. Symphony no. 3 in C minor Op 78 (the Organ Symphony) 4th Movement Maestoso. www.youtube.com/watch?v=Xnhhw85zK2I&list=RD02hopaQjQFUYw [accessed 16 January 2014].

15. General Medical Council. *Treatment and Care towards the End of Life: good practice in decision making.* London: GMC, 2010, www.gmc-uk.org/End_of_life.pdf_32486688.pdf [accessed 16 January 2014].

16. Aristotle. *Ethics,* Books VIII and IX.

17. Aristotle. *Ethics,* Book X.

18. Works by Aristotle include the *Physics, De Anima,* several seminal works on logic as well as the *Ethics* and the *Politics.*

19. Whitehead AN. *Process and Reality* (eds DR Griffin, DW Sherburne). New York: Free Press, 1978 [1929], http://heidigustafson.com/wp-content/uploads/2012/07/11953-process_and_reality_an.pdf [accessed 4 March 2014].

20. McNab A. On the shoulders of giants. 2001. www.isaacnewton.org.uk/essays/Giants [accessed 16 January 2014].

21. Doyal L, Gough I. *A Theory of Human Need.* London: Macmillan Education, 1991.

22. World Health Organization. Frequently asked questions: what is the WHO definition of health? 2103. www.who.int/suggestions/faq/en/index.html [accessed 16 January 2014].

23. World Health Organization. Mental health: a state of well-being. 2013. www.who.int/features/factfiles/mental_health/en [accessed 4 March 2014].

24. Huber M. How should we define health? *British Medical Journal* 2011; **343**: d4163. dx.doi.org/10.1136/bmj.d4163.

25. Toon PD. *What is Good General Practice?* (Occasional Paper 65). London: RCGP, 1994.

26. Hart JT. *A New Kind of Doctor.* London: Merlin Press, 1988.

27. Kramer G. Payment for Performance and the QOF: are we doing the right thing? *British Journal of General Practice* 2012; **62(596)**: e217–19, doi: 10.3399/bjgp12X630151.

28. Hanrath P. Contribution to Autumn Colloquium on the question 'What values should underlie our out of hours health service?' LinkedIn Primary Care Ethics Forum 2013. www.linkedin.com/groupItem?view=&gid=4315768&type=member&item=269149590&qid=08b678b4-b9e2-483e-9c05-d3591a635295&trk=groups_most_recent-0-b-cmr&gobac k=%2Eanp_4315768_1382092285278_1%2Egmr_4315768 [accessed 8 July 2014].

29. Sontag S. *Illness as Metaphor.* New York: Vintage Books, 1979.

30. Prostate Cancer UK. PSA test. 2012. http://prostatecanceruk.org/information/diagnosis/diagnosis-tests/psa-test [accessed 16 January 2014].

31. Dr Iona Heath during workshop on prevention and anticipatory care. WONCA, Paris, 2007.

32. Prof. Sir Mike Rawlins at the RCGP Annual Conference, Liverpool, 20–22 October 2011.

33. Dr David Haslam at the RSM Primary Care Ethics Conference, London, 20 February 2013.

34. Sackett DL, Rosenberg WM, Gray JA, *et al.* Evidence based medicine: what it is and what it isn't. *British Medical Journal* 1996; **312(7023)**: 71–2, www.ncbi.nlm.nih.gov/pmc/articles/PMC2349778/pdf/bmj00524-0009.pdf [accessed 16 January 2014].

35. Balint M. *The Doctor, His Patient and the Illness* (2nd edn). London: Churchill Livingstone, 1964 [1957].

36. Propp V. *Morphology of the Folktale* (2nd edn, rev. and ed. LA Wagner). Austin, TX: University of Texas Press, 1968.

37. Lefcourt HM. *Locus of Control: current trends in theory and research* (2nd edn). New Jersey: Lawrence Erlbaum Associates, 1982.

38. Just three of the thirty-six dramatic situations identified by Goethe, described in G Polti. *The Thirty-Six Dramatic Situations.* Trans. L Ray. Franklin, OH: James Knapp Reeve, 1921, http://archive.org/stream/thirtysixdramati00poltuoft/thirtysixdramati00poltuoft_djvu.txt [accessed 16 January 2014].

39. Aristotle. *Ethics*, Books VII and IX.

40. Aristotle. *The Politics* (trans. TA Sinclair 1962, rev. TJ Saunders). Harmondsworth: Penguin, 1981.

41. Quotation from Harry Lime in the film *The Third Man* (1949): 'in Italy for 30 years under the Borgias they had warfare, terror, murder, and bloodshed, but they produced Michelangelo, Leonardo da Vinci, and the Renaissance. In Switzerland they had brotherly love – they had 500 years of democracy and peace, and what did that produce? The cuckoo clock.'

42. Lewis CS. *The Four Loves*. London: Collins, 1960, https://thepathtolight.com/uploads/c.s._lewis_-_the_four_loves__christian_library_.pdf [accessed 16 January 2014].

43. Aristotle. *Ethics*, Book X.

44. Balint. *The Doctor, His Patient and the Illness* (*op. cit.*).

45. Jacobs D. A good doctor-patient relationship creates a strong placebo effect. 2013. www.placeboeffect.com/doctor-patient-relationship [accessed 16 January 2014].

46. Balint. *The Doctor, His Patient and the Illness* (*op. cit.*).

47. Heath I. *The Mystery of General Practice*. London: Nuffield Provincial Hospitals Trust, 1995, www.nuffieldtrust.org.uk/sites/files/nuffield/publication/The_Mystery_of_General_Practice.pdf [accessed 16 January 2014].

48. Dante A. *The Divine Comedy: Inferno*. Trans. HF Carey. London: Cassell, 1892, www.gutenberg.org/files/8800/8800-h/files/8789/8789-h/p1.htm [accessed 16 January 2014]. The opening lines of Canto I:

    In the midway of this our mortal life
    I found me in a gloomy wood, astray
    Gone from the path direct

49. Heath. *The Mystery of General Practice* (*op. cit.*).

50. Julian P. Being there. In: A Elder, O Samuel (eds), *While I'm Here, Doctor*. London: Tavistock/Routledge, 1987, pp. 77–83.

51. Sir Lawrence Alma-Tadema's *Portrait of Dr Washington Epps, My Doctor*. Carnegie Museum of Art, Pittsburgh, USA, May 1885, www.topofart.com/artists/Sir_Lawrence_Alma-Tadema/painting/5970/Portrait_of_Dr_Washington_Epps,_My_Doctor.php [accessed 16 January 2014].

52. These are imaginary cases, although like most GPs I have encountered many like these over the years.

53. Neighbour R. *The Inner Consultation*. Dordrecht, Netherlands: Kluwer Academic Publishers Group, 1987.

54. Macintyre A. *After Virtue: a study in moral theory* (2nd edn). London: Duckworth, 1985.

55. *The Rule of St Benedict in English* (ed. T Fry). Minnesota: Liturgical Press, 1982, Chapter 48. Another translation is available at: www.osb.org/rb/text/rbemjo3.html#48 [accessed 16 January 2014].

56. Aristotle. *Ethics*, Book X.

57. Nussbaum MC, Sen A. *The Quality of Life*. Oxford: Clarendon Press, 1993.

Chapter 4

Concepts of disease and a narrative of flourishing

In the last chapter we explored the implications of seeing health care as a MacIntyrean practice for our understanding of its nature and purpose. We examined the concept of flourishing and how participating in health care as a patient might contribute to flourishing. In this chapter we will look at the nature and purpose of health care from another perspective, by examining the boundaries of illness and disease and their biomedical treatment.

There have been interminable discussions about the words 'illness' and 'disease', and I don't intend to contribute to this debate, which is largely a matter of semantics. By illness I mean a state opposed to wellness; a move to what Susan Sontag calls 'the kingdom of the sick'.[1] This has mostly negative consequences, but citizens of the kingdom of the sick do have certain privileges. They are not held responsible for their condition and its consequences; they get sympathy rather than blame and are cared for. They are excused from work and social responsibilities, and there are also financial and other benefits awarded to those who are ill or incapacitated.[2]

By disease I mean a diagnostic category based on medical (and sometimes psychological) understanding of symptom patterns and pathophysiology. These categories are used as intervening variables between the experiences of a person who is, or who believes himself to be, ill and prognosis and treatment – usually although not always in biomedical terms. Seeing a person as ill means defining a group of features (physical characteristics, experiences, behaviours or functional limitations) as part of a disease and separating them from the person who 'has' the disease.[3]

Although the factual classification of diseases and the evaluation of a condition as an illness are logically separate, we do not usually separate them in everyday usage. Most diagnostic disease categories are illnesses (although in general practice we often use categories such as 'not an illness' or 'not X-disease'). Having a disease means you are ill. There are a few diagnostic categories that are not illnesses (Gilbert's syndrome and racial neutropenia are examples) but these are only described because they may be confused with other diagnostic categories that are evaluated as illnesses. Debates about the boundaries of a disease are sometimes factual debates about where the data suggest it makes sense to draw a line. More often however they are really evaluative debates about the boundary between illness and wellness, although participants in those debates often think they are discussing factual issues, and may attempt to use empirical evidence to support their case.

There is now a consensus that illness, and therefore the classification of disease categories as illnesses, is evaluative.[4] Attempts by Kendell[5] and Scadding and colleagues[6] in the 1970s to define disease on a value-free basis were generally seen as unsuccessful. In a world of pluralist values and competing ethical frameworks, divisions between health and illness often seem to be arbitrary and variable, based on relativist or emotivist views of values, or are disputed because of differing concepts of the proper role of medicine.

Although there has been little discussion on the general nature of illness and disease in the academic literature in recent years, there are heated debates in both popular and medical media about specific conditions. There are arguments about whether conditions should be seen as diseases at all (for example attention deficit hyperactivity disorder (ADHD), social anxiety disorder, alcoholism, drug dependency). Many diseases have unclear causes and there are different views on these (for example chronic fatigue syndrome/myalgic encephalitis [ME]). Many diseases have fuzzy edges, and there are debates about when biomedical treatment is appropriate (for example depression, hypertension, hyperlipidaemia or obesity). Views about whether procedures such as breast reduction, Botox injections, drugs for erectile dysfunction and surgery for varicose veins should be available on the NHS also depend mostly on whether we see the problems they address as 'real' illnesses or not. Most of these debates arise from different evaluations of the conditions, although this is not always accepted and different views are often argued in terms of 'the evidence'.

In this chapter I will discuss some of these contested areas to try to understand the underlying causes of these disputes in terms of the fragmented moral discourse MacIntyre describes, and to see whether a MacIntyrean virtue ethic can help us formulate some general principles (perhaps what Hursthouse would call 'v-rules')[7] on how to define the boundary between illness and the person.

What is depression?

Depression is a good example of a contested condition. It is a common problem encountered every day in general practice, and is interesting because there has recently been a major shift in attitudes. For some years there was much talk of depression being 'missed' by GPs. For instance, a consensus statement published in the *British Medical Journal* in 1992 suggested that 'at any consultation about half the patients consulting with depression are not recognised. A further 10% are recognised at subsequent consultations, and 20% remit during this time, but the remaining 20% may remain unrecognised even after six months.'[8]

General practitioners were encouraged to be more aware of hidden depression, particularly when it presented with somatic symptoms, and to use screening tools to identify it.

To some extent this still goes on; for example the Quality and Outcomes Framework (QOF) payment system for GPs includes points for screening patients with chronic diseases for depression. But in the last decade the rate of diagnosis and treatment of depression has risen sharply, and the pendulum has swung the other way, so that some commentators are now saying depression is over-diagnosed and unhappiness is being medicalised.[9]

One reason for these different views is that the boundary between depression and unhappiness is fuzzy. Depression is not unique in this. Other disease categories defined on the basis of a continuous variable – for example diabetes and hypertension – are fuzzy too. When a disease is defined on a categorical variable the boundary is clear – you can't be a bit pregnant, or have a touch of bubonic plague. But when a disease is defined on a continuous variable the normal and the abnormal merge imperceptibly into each other, so the boundary is to some extent arbitrary. A few people are obviously depressed; most are not. But there are some in the middle where it is hard to decide whether they are depressed or just transitorily unhappy. A line must be drawn between normal and abnormal values, and you can just meet or just miss the diagnostic criterion wherever that line is drawn.

Depression is a psychological rather than a physical concept, and the problems of measurement in psychology are often trickier than in physiology, so it is harder to find a reliable measuring instrument. More importantly, however, depression is a complex concept; the Patient Health Questionnaire (PHQ9) tool commonly used to quantify depression in general practice is based on nine symptoms.[10] The more variables involved in defining a condition, the fuzzier its edges. This problem affects disease categories defined on physiological as well as psychological criteria. Diabetes is a physiological concept essentially defined in terms of one measurement – fasting blood glucose. Metabolic syndrome is also a physiological concept, but it is fuzzier than diabetes because like depression it is defined in terms of several variables. Rheumatology is full of complex fuzzy categories defined largely in physiological terms.

Stability of measures over time is important too: fasting blood sugar is fairly stable, but resting blood pressure is not. Mood can fluctuate wildly and rapidly. Some measures of depression, for example the PHQ9, try to achieve stability by asking for a self-assessment over a period of time, Others, for example the Beck Depression Inventory, are 'snapshots'. Here all the questions are in the present tense and no timeframe is specified, encouraging the respondent to examine her feelings and thoughts at the moment of completing the questionnaire.[11]

So some uncertainties about the limits of depression are empirical problems of setting boundaries and making measurements. These problems are common throughout the biological sciences, and are essentially similar to the difficulties that sometimes occur in placing a plant or animal in a particular species or family, or in deciding the relationships between different phyla and kingdoms.

But the problem is also evaluative, and can be seen as another example of the moral fragmentation MacIntyre describes, although the fragments are not the same as those discussed in Chapter 1.

The drifting fragments – normality

Some people see a condition as an illness because it is statistically abnormal; for example Parker's argument that depression is normal based on population surveys[12] relies on this assumption. Another normative view sees a disease not as a statistical deviation, but as a deviation from a sort of 'platonic form' of normality. The healthy person has certain characteristics, and if most of the population fall short of this ideal then they are all ill. This concept underlies the World Health Organization's definition of health as 'a state of complete physical and mental wellbeing'.[13] Fulford's concept of disease as 'action failure',[14] the inability to do something one ought to be able to do, may also be based on this premise.

Definitions based on these normative assumptions are sometimes criticised as oppressive, pathologising those whose only problem is that they differ from the majority or do not conform to a social norm. In 1973 homosexuality was removed from the *Diagnostic and Statistical Manual of Mental Disorders* (DSM)[15] on the basis of this argument. The same argument has recently been used by those opposed to treating people with Asperger's syndrome as disordered,[16,17] and with regard to dyslexia[18] and intersex.[19] In this view those with these conditions are not 'disabled' but 'differently-abled'.

The dualist fragment

It is sometimes felt that an identifiable physical basis justifies the classification of a condition as an illness. For example much heat is generated between those who believe chronic fatigue syndrome to be the result of a viral infection and those who are agnostic as to its cause or think it may be psychogenic. Those who hold the former view tend to prefer the term 'ME', which emphasises its physical cause. This seems to be based on a dualist view of human nature, in which diseases belong on the physical side of the mind–body divide, whilst aspects of the person lie in the mental sphere. Real illnesses have their basis in physiological processes; imagined illnesses are 'all in the mind'.

Much of the difficulty with mental illness stems from this, because even more obviously than physical illness, it is 'all in the mind'. In fact as Fulford[20] points out most of the symptoms of physical illness are in the mind too; pain and other unpleasant sensations are experienced in the mind, though attributed to causes in the body. Even our experience of loss of function depends on a mental assessment of what we ought to be able to do.

As our understanding of the genetics and physiology of human nature and diversity expands (particularly recently our knowledge of neurophysiology and genetics) we have an identifiable physical cause for conditions – for example shyness[21] – that were previously inexplicable, or which could only be understood in psychological terms. From the dualist perspective this moves them from being part of the person into being diseases. Thus personhood becomes the ontological equivalent of the 'God of the gaps';[22] as we understand more about the physiological underpinning of our humanity, fewer of the problems we face are part of that humanity and more are reified as 'diseases'. Also, however, as we gain this understanding, which shows how closely mind and body are intertwined, a dualist mind–body division become increasingly untenable.

The consequentialist fragment

For those clinging to the consequentialist fragment of the moral shipwreck, suffering is necessarily bad, and any action that decreases suffering or prolongs life morally right. Life is a succession of good and bad experiences, beads of different shapes and colours strung together on the thread of existence. Ugly and broken beads need to be repaired or replaced as quickly as possible in the easiest way available. From this perspective it doesn't matter whether depression is statistically abnormal or a deviation from an ideal state, or whether it is based in the mind or in the body. All that matters is whether taking the tablets reduces suffering and increases pleasure. And all means of removing suffering are equally valid; the only significant differences between drug treatment and psychotherapy are efficacy and cost. In this view there is no place for negative experiences with positive outcomes, other than those (for example surgery) that substitute short-term pain for long-term gain.

From this perspective the distinction between illnesses, risk factors and prodromal stages of conditions that may lead to illness if untreated is irrelevant, which is perhaps why it is sometimes blurred in practice. Hyperlipidaemia, mild and moderate hypertension, chronic kidney disease (CKD) stages 2 and 3, and early cervical intracellular neoplasia are asymptomatic conditions or risk factors that may or may not progress to overt illness which we detect and treat. But because modifying them reduces the risk of progression to illness, it makes good consequentialist sense to screen for and treat them if it leads to the greater good of the greatest number.

Although for consequentialist gain screening programmes do not need to distinguish between a disease that is also an illness and a risk factor that is not yet an illness, the diagnosis and treatment of a risk factor can be seen as implying a transfer to the kingdom of the ill. Chronic kidney 'disease' is a good example of this.[23] The term is used for all levels of renal function; stage 1 is completely satisfactory and stage 2 is mild impairment for which no action is needed. Only at stage 3 (which is still asymptomatic) is the risk of progression to symptomatic renal impairment high enough to consider intervention to slow deterioration, and only stages 4 or 5 have an impact on wellbeing that we might properly call illness. But patients are often alarmed when told that they have CKD stage 3, even though it just means they have an increased risk of renal failure in the future, perhaps because in other conditions they may have heard of stage 3 as being quite advanced. It can be hard to reassure them that, because the rate of deterioration is usually slow and predictable, problems lie in the distant future and may never occur.

Disease-mongering

A new treatment often triggers the treatment of risk factors, the definition of new diseases or an increase in rates of diagnosis of existing ones (which is essentially the same because it means classifying as diseased people who previously would have been considered normal). It can be argued that this is a desirable response to new opportunities – there is after all little point in identifying problems one can do nothing about. Others see it as 'disease-mongering'[24] – a dangerous trend for a pharmaceutical industry motivated by a drive for profits to create markets by pathologising conditions formerly accepted as normal risks or part of human experience.

Wolinsky considers the increased diagnosis and treatment of conditions as varied as metabolic syndrome, osteoporosis, ADHD and social phobia as examples of this phenomenon.[25] The organisation 'Drugwatch'[26] argues that it is an essential part of seeing health care as a business, controlled by market forces, citing a number of specific examples, whereas drug companies argue that they are merely promoting 'disease awareness'.[27]

Whatever the rights and wrongs of particular instances, seeing health care as a practice whose purpose is the cultivation of the virtues and the creation of its internal goods to promote human flourishing rather than as a means of profit is an important defence against inappropriate medicalisation.

Illness and responsibility

There is however another reason why conditions such as social phobia and attention deficit disorder may be classified as illnesses rather than personality characteristics, which is the link between illness and responsibility. Defining a problem as a disease implies that it is involuntary, and therefore outside the range of things for which we can be held responsible. It is an 'excusing factor'[28] for behaviour or inability to perform. The argument runs like this:

My behaviour is the result of my illness or *I can't do that because of my illness.*

My illness is not my fault.

Therefore it follows that;

My behaviour is not my fault or *It's not my fault I can't do that.*

Usually the excusing aspect of an illness is secondary to the classification of a condition as an illness on other grounds; psychoanalysts often refer to this excusing as 'secondary' gain; but sometimes it is the main reason for defining a condition as an illness. We want to feel sympathy for the person with the condition rather than blame him, so we decide he must be ill. The logic flows in the other direction:

His behaviour shouldn't be seen as his fault.

Behaviour resulting from an illness is not his fault.

Therefore:

His behaviour must be the result of an illness.

This logic however only works if the first premise is accepted. Even when a condition is statistically or normatively abnormal, can be understood in biomedical terms, has an effective treatment that relieves suffering, or can be profitably treated, if it does not attract sympathy then the effect of the definition on responsibility and its excusing implications may make its definition as a disease controversial. Some people may argue:

His behaviour is his fault.

Behaviour resulting from an illness is not his fault.

Therefore:

His behaviour cannot be the result of an illness.

There are many examples of this. The treatment of alcoholism as a disease is well established but continues to provoke controversy;[29] other forms of drug addiction are sometimes treated as diseases, sometimes as crimes,[30] and the continuance of this debate in popular[31] as well as academic fora is a good example of the interminable nature of moral arguments based on disconnected moral fragments.

There is even more scepticism about the extension of the disease view of addiction to other conditions – for example sex addiction. The case of US President Bill Clinton illustrates some of the arguments. When his relationship with Monica Lewinsky became public there was discussion in the press as to whether he was a sex addict, and whether this was because he had an alcoholic father.[32] Others however argued that 'sex addiction' does not exist but is 'an attempt to avoid responsibility by medicalizing misbehaviour'.[33] More recently a study of brain responses in sexually aroused people has been interpreted as evidence that sex addiction is nothing more than strong sexual desire, and that 'Philanderers may need a new excuse for extramarital affairs'.[34]

The status of other conditions defined mainly in terms of socially unacceptable patterns of behaviour are also controversial. Is ADHD a neurological disease, a habit of behaving badly or an example of the huge variation in human nature, some of which society finds it hard to cope with?[35]

Illness is defined in a social context. Value systems are inherent in medicine. With adult attention deficit disorder, some people whose brains are easily distracted are [annoyed] at being labelled [and] will say that they are just high energy and creative; others will be thankful they were diagnosed, treated and had their attention span restored to almost normal.[36]

Similarly Asperger's syndrome may be defined as a disease because it is a deviation from a platonic norm of human functioning or on consequentialist grounds; conversely it may be evaluated as a part of who someone is, and welcomed as a contribution to human diversity.

Self-inflicted illness

Even when the status as diseases of conditions is less controversial, there is sometimes a feeling that deliberate actions by the person affected caused their condition, and that therefore they are responsible for it and they should not be treated at public expense. Is obesity a self-inflicted problem caused by over-eating and lack of exercise (the vices of gluttony and sloth), or a misfortune resulting from a poor upbringing, an industry that pushes unhealthy food and poverty that makes healthy choices unaffordable? And are external treatments such as drug therapy or bariatric surgery appropriate, or should those affected just eat less and exercise more? Smokers with lung cancer, skiers with fractures, and people contracting HIV infection through promiscuous sex are other situations where similar arguments are sometimes made.

Low-priority procedures

These differences of opinion can have practical importance, leading to policies about whether a particular condition should be treated on the NHS at public expense. A recent move in health policy has been attempts to control NHS budgets by limiting medical intervention in 'low priority procedures'.[37] Sometimes the argument is that there is little or no evidence of benefit from the procedure, so that it is not good value for money. Tonsillectomy for many cases of sore throat is an example of this.[38] This is an empirical judgement made on the basis of evidence, and has no evaluative implications about the condition.

In other cases, however, the choice of restricted treatments reflects a view that they lie outside the proper limits of health care, based on evaluative assumptions rather than empirical judgements on cost and benefit. Surgery primarily for aesthetic reasons such as treatment for acne scarring, body contouring procedures, breast augmentation and reduction (with exceptions when large breasts cause pain) are examples of this.

Although the underlying values are rarely made explicit, there seems to be a distinction made between correction of defects and enhancement of the norm. As Harris[39] points out, the boundary between the two is hazy because the norm has fuzzy edges. De Sousa[40] reminds us that aesthetic improvement is often seen as personal vanity, or a lamentable submission to the superficial priority placed on appearance in our society, which public funds should not support. There also seems to be a distinction made between improving personal appearance by exercise or diet (laudable activities) and achieving the same result by surgical intervention (taking the easy way out), perhaps arising from a value system that is a mixture of puritanism and the British stiff upper lip. Consequentialists are of course unimpressed by such distinctions.

Paying for treatment

Most prescription charge exemption criteria (age, disability, benefit criteria, pregnancy, etc.) seem to be rough and ready attempts to protect the vulnerable from being deprived of medication they can't afford. But there is also a list of diseases[41] that exempt those diagnosed from these charges:

a permanent fistula (for example caecostomy, colostomy, laryngostomy or ileostomy) requiring an appliance or continuous surgical dressing

a form of hypoadrenalism (for example Addison's disease) for which specific substitution therapy is needed

diabetes insipidus or other forms of hypopituitarism

diabetes mellitus, except where treatment is by diet alone

hypoparathyroidism

myasthenia gravis

myxoedema (hypothyroidism requiring thyroid hormone replacement)

epilepsy requiring continuous anticonvulsive therapy[42]

Why conditions are placed on this list is not obvious. Although they are all chronic conditions, this is not the justification, because some common chronic diseases such as asthma and heart disease are not included. Many of the conditions involve replacement of a substance normally produced by the body without which life is not possible (Addison's disease, hypothyroidism, hypoparathyroidism, myasthenia gravis, diabetes insipidus). Diabetes mellitus is also on the list, although these days most diabetic patients are treated with oral hypoglycaemic drugs. When, however, the list was drawn up treatment for diabetes usually meant insulin replacement, another example of replacing a substance that is normally naturally produced. Perhaps therefore there was an implicit distinction between replacing substances needed to sustain life and drugs needed to treat disease, akin to the distinction between ordinary and extraordinary means?

This hypothesis does not however explain the inclusion of those with permanent fistulae and epilepsy, nor why it is not specific drugs used to treat those conditions that are exempt from prescription charges (as contraceptives are as a matter of public policy, whether or not the person concerned would otherwise pay a charge). The exemption covers all medication for the person with the condition.

The arrangements regarding drug treatments for erectile dysfunction on the NHS are similarly illogical. The introduction of safe, acceptable and effective oral treatment for this condition produced enormous anxiety amongst those responsible for NHS funding. It was feared that the demand for better erections and hence the cost involved might overwhelm NHS budgets. It was therefore decided to breach the principle that all prescribable drugs are available on NHS prescription to NHS patients, The NHS only pays for drugs for erectile dysfunction[43] when the patient has one of a number of chronic diseases where impotence is common. All other patients must have a private prescription and pay for the drugs.

Is this because the first group is seen as having a physical basis lacking in the latter, or that idiopathic impotence is seen as part of normal variation and its pharmacological correction as enhancement, whereas when it is part of a chronic disease process it is seen as a defect meriting therapy? Or perhaps this is a sort of 'grandfather clause' that allows free prescriptions of the newer drugs for those who might previously have been treated with the rather unpleasant and invasive injectable drugs for erectile dysfunction? Perhaps these were mostly prescribed for patients whose impotence resulted from a known disease, whilst patients who presented with 'functional impotence' would be more likely to be offered psychological treatment rather than intra-penile injections? One also cannot help wondering whether unconscious puritanism plays a part, particularly in view of the guidance that where NHS prescriptions are allowed these should be limited to four doses per month.

Anxieties about cost control clearly play a part in these decisions, because NHS-funded medical interventions are not always related to a disease. Menstruation is a normal function, but it is commonplace to give medication on the NHS to postpone a period when it appears likely to come at an inappropriate time, for example for a wedding or a romantic holiday. However, here the drugs involved are cheap and the numbers asking for this treatment insufficient to threaten NHS budgets.

But distinctions between what the NHS pays for and what is excluded cannot always be explained in terms of costs. The prevention of infectious disease amongst travellers abroad demonstrates similar apparently arbitrary distinctions. Where defined indications are met, protection by immunisation against typhoid, cholera, rabies, yellow fever, hepatitis A, etc. is provided and administered without charge to NHS patients. But NHS patients must have a private prescription for malaria prophylaxis by taking tablets, even when official guidance is that this is necessary.

What is the logic behind this distinction? Some courses of malaria prophylaxis are cheaper than some immunisations. The cost of treating a case of imported malaria cannot be predictably less than the cost of a case of imported typhoid or cholera; in fact the overall cost may be higher, as imported malaria is commoner than imported cases of the other diseases. Exact figures vary of course and precisely comparable data are not readily available, but the data[44–46] suggest the order of magnitude is about 1500 cases of malaria, 200 cases of typhoid and ten cases of cholera per year. An economic argument does not therefore seem sustainable.

There would be a public health case for preferentially funding the prevention of diseases such as typhoid or cholera that could be transmitted within the UK – but this is not generally the case either with rabies, for which immunisation of those at risk is free, or malaria, for which patients have to pay. (I have been told that there is a remote possibility that malaria could re-establish itself in a population of mosquitoes living in the marshes around the Thames Estuary, but it seems unlikely that this theoretical risk is affecting policy.)

Perhaps this reminds us that we cannot always expect to find a logical, even if implicit, rationale behind NHS policy. The influence of pressure groups and the personal sympathies of those drawing up regulations may produce a policy based on expediency rather than reason.

Summary of our understanding of the debates about disease categories

On the basis of the account of the uses of the concept of disease discussed above, I would suggest that a typical disease category fulfils five criteria:

1. It is a set of features of an individual – experiences, appearances, behaviours and functional limitations, including decreased life expectancy – associated with pain, disability or some other type of distress.

2. These features have a common cause that can be understood in biomedical terms, and for which a biomedical treatment is the most appropriate course of action.

3. Having these features is both 'platonically' and statistically abnormal – they mark a deviation from the ideal human form, and are not shared with the vast majority of human beings.

4. It is qualitatively different from 'normality' – a line can easily be drawn between those who fall into the category and those who don't.

5. The cause of the condition is clearly outside the control of the individual involved, and so she cannot be held responsible for them.

I would suggest that when a condition obviously fulfils all these criteria there is rarely any debate about its status as a disease and whether or not it should be treated at the public expense. This is for example the case with conditions such as myocardial infarction, most cancers, accidental injury, and infections such as pneumonia and gastroenteritis.

Disputes however arise when only some of the criteria are fulfilled or only partly fulfilled, or where there are different opinions as to whether a criterion is fulfilled. Thus people disagree about whether Asperger's syndrome, homosexuality and intersex are disabilities or not. Alcoholism and other addictions are clearly platonically and statistically abnormal, but it is not agreed whether or not they are beyond the control of the individual concerned.

There may be differences of opinion on more than one criterion. For example, people may disagree about whether a large nose or breasts cause pain, disability or distress for which a biomedical (surgical) treatment is appropriate, whether the problem is better seen as a mental health problem of subjective body image or as an instance of vice of vanity that is not a matter for health care. They may also disagree on where the line between the normal and the abnormal nose or breast lies.

Disease and illness in a MacIntyrean world

This is only a partial and superficial analysis of the implicit values we bring to deciding whether conditions should be considered as diseases and treated at the public expense. However, it illustrates that, as with other aspects of health care, disputes reflect implicit and often unacknowledged values, and that differences of opinion arise at least in part from a fragmented moral discourse. How might a MacIntyrean approach affect our view?

First it would affect our willingness to define a state as a disease. The heart of MacIntyre's thesis is that we need to see life as a narrative unity in which the cultivation of the virtues leads to a flourishing narrative. The definition of an aspect of our being as a disease on whatever grounds separates it from our personhood. It therefore follows that, unless this is the only way in which we can flourish, we should seek to integrate aspects of our life into our personhood and our narrative rather than externalise them, because removing aspects of our experience from our personhood diminishes the richness of the narrative.

This means we will be unwilling to define conditions as illnesses on grounds of a platonic norm, because human diversity is something to celebrate rather than to eradicate. We therefore might favour helping those with Asperger's syndrome or ADHD to flourish with their condition rather than normalise it with drugs. One way in which this can be done is through the hermeneutic or interpretative function, helping people understand and make sense of what is happening to them rather than trying to change it. As Heath has pointed out, the 'gatekeeper' role of the GP includes not only keeping the gate between primary and secondary care, but also the gate between health and illness. This is an important part of the interpretative function, which as discussed in the last chapter lies at the heart of a MacIntyrean approach to health care as a practice.

It may also affect our attitude to treatment. For both normalists and consequentialists a disease is something to be got rid of in the most effective and cheapest way possible. Both groups are pragmatists. The only difference between different drug and psychological therapies is how well and how cheaply they do the job. For the MacIntyrean, however, it is not enough to abolish symptoms and improve functioning in any way possible; this should be done in the way that best contributes to flourishing. This implies that we should favour treatments that promote autonomy not as a right to be protected but as a capacity to be enhanced. Thus for example in depression psychological approaches that enhance the individual's capacity to overcome challenges may be seen as preferable to drug treatments where the individual is a passive participant; flourishing is usually enhanced by narratives in which the patient is a hero rather than a victim. This does not mean that drug treatments for depression have no place; like staking a plant they may provide the external support necessary for growth to full potential. Patients may need to be helped to overcome their depression by drugs before they are in a condition to benefit from psychological treatments, in the same way that healing a broken limb requires it to be externally supported in a plaster cast at first but later actively strengthened by physiotherapeutic exercises.

Illness becomes part of life's narrative rather than an interruption to it. Approaches to illness that help someone grow in virtue and enhance the fullness of their humanity as a result of their illness (what Maslow calls self-actualisation[47] and St Paul calls attaining the measure of the fullness of the stature of Christ)[48] are in general to be preferred to treatments that leave the patient where he was, or worse that increase dependency. Again this may have significant effects on how we practise health care.

It also follows that how we define illness and disease will rightly vary between individuals, because every individual's flourishing narrative is unique. Recent emphasis on evidence-based practice has led to increasing use of guidelines, care pathways and protocols that rely on standard definitions of disease categories and treatment interventions. Whilst it make sense to treat people according to the best available evidence, the MacIntyrean would argue that this needs to include the particular evidence relating to that specific individual, as well as general evidence derived from studies in which all patients in a defined category are treated similarly. Over-emphasis on the importance of general rather than particular evidence risks ignoring individual differences. This perspective will probably lead to more variation in treatment than would flow from a consequentialist perspective, not as a result of the consumerist ideal of patient choice but because flourishing may be best achieved in different ways for different people, and the patient and the clinician work out in collaboration what this is for each individual.

Finally it implies defining the medical role in functional rather than ontological terms. Whether or not a condition fits the criteria for being a disease matters less than whether medical intervention can contribute to flourishing. Thus from this perspective the postponement of menstruation for a wedding or a holiday discussed above is justified; this is not because it is the treatment of a disease, but because such celebrations and ceremonies are important contributors to flourishing, and a course of norethisterone can modify the patient's narrative to make it more flourishing. Because a certain level of medical expertise is needed to check for contraindications, discuss side effects, etc. before taking the treatment, this is appropriately done by a doctor even though no illness is involved.

Conclusion

In this and the previous chapter we have seen a little of how the experience of patients in health care is confused and distorted by the moral fragmentation of the world in which we live, and some of the implications of seeing health care as a practice devoted to promoting flourishing through the cultivation of the virtues. Our next task is to consider the impact of seeing healthcare in MacIntyrean terms for the other main group involved in it, the professionals. Because I am a general practitioner I will discuss this mostly in terms of the impact on general practitioners. Although many of the arguments apply equally to other doctors, to nurses, other clinicians and healthcare managers, I have neither the space nor the experience to discuss these; this will be for others better qualified in those areas to do.

Notes

1. Sontag S. *Illness as Metaphor.* New York: Vintage Books, 1979.

2. Toon PD. *Towards a Philosophy of General Practice* (Occasional Paper 78). London: RCGP, 1998.

3. For a fuller discussion, see Toon. *Towards a Philosophy of General Practice.*

4. Toon PD. Defining 'disease': classification must be distinguished from evaluation. *Journal of Medical Ethics* 1981; **7(4)**: 197–201.

5. Kendell RE. The concept of disease and its implications for psychiatry. *British Journal of Psychiatry* 1975; **127**: 305–15, http://bjp.rcpsych.org/content/127/4/305.short [accessed 16 January 2014].

6. Scadding JG. Health and disease: what can medicine do for philosophy? *Journal of Medical Ethics* 1988; **14(3)**: 118–24.

7. Hursthouse R. *On Virtue Ethics.* Oxford: Oxford University Press, 1999.

8. Paykel ES, Priest RG. Recognition and management of depression in general practice: consensus statement. *British Medical Journal* 1992; **305(6863)**: 1198, www.bmj.com/content/305/6863/1198 [accessed 16 January 2014].

9. Parker G. Is depression overdiagnosed? Yes. *British Medical Journal* 2007; **335**: 328, www.bmj.com/content/335/7615/328 [accessed 16 January 2014].

10. Willacy H. Patient Health Questionnaire (PHQ-9). 2013. www.patient.co.uk/doctor/patient-health-questionnaire-phq-9 [accessed 4 March 2014].

11. Beck AT. Beck's Depression Inventory. 1961. http://drjeremybarowsky.com/site/wp-content/uploads/2013/07/JB_Assessment-Tools_Depression_07_17_13.pdf [accessed 4 March 2014].

12. Parker. Is depression overdiagnosed? (*op. cit.*)

13. World Health Organization. *Constitution of the World Health Organization.* Basic Documents, 45th edition, Supplement, October 2006, www.who.int/governance/eb/who_constitution_en.pdf [accessed 16 January 2014].

14. Fulford KWM. *Moral Theory and Medical Practice.* Cambridge: Cambridge University Press, 1989.

15. Herek GM. Facts about homosexuality and mental health. 2012. http://psychology.ucdavis.edu/rainbow/html/facts_mental_health.html [accessed 16 January 2014].

16. Asperger's Syndrome is Not Necessarily a Disorder. Discussion started on 28 August 2009 on Wrongplanet.net – the online resource and community for autism and Asperger's. www.wrongplanet.net/postt136245.html [accessed 16 January 2014].

17. Saner E. It is not a disease, it is a way of life. *Guardian,* 7 August 2007, www.guardian.co.uk/society/2007/aug/07/health.medicineandhealth [accessed 16 January 2014].

18. Foster C. My son is dyslexic, and I'm glad. 2011. http://blog.practicalethics.ox.ac.uk/2011/10/my-sons-dyslexic-and-im-glad [accessed 16 January 2014].

19. Reis E. Divergence or disorder? The politics of naming intersex. *Perspectives in Biology and Medicine* 2007; **50(4)**: 535–43, www.academia.edu/1172243/_Divergence_or_Disorder_The_Politics_of_Naming_Intersex_ [accessed 16 January 2014].

20. Fulford. *Moral Theory and Medical Practice* (*op. cit.*).

21. Cunningham A. Social phobia or just shyness? 2002. http://serendip.brynmawr.edu/bb/neuro/neuro02/web3/acunningham.html [accessed 16 January 2014].

22. Are gaps in scientific knowledge evidence for God? *BioLogos*. 2013. http://biologos.org/questions/god-of-the-gaps [accessed 16 January 2014].

23. Renal Association. CKD stages. www.renal.org/whatwedo/InformationResources/CKDegUIDE/CKDstages.aspx [accessed 16 January 2014].

24. Moynihan R, Heath I, Henry D. Selling sickness: the pharmaceutical industry and disease mongering. *British Medical Journal* 2002; **324(7342)**: 886–91, www.bmj.com/cgi/content/full/324/7342/886#art [accessed 16 January 2014].

25. Wolinsky H. Disease mongering and drug marketing. Does the pharmaceutical industry manufacture diseases as well as drugs? *EMBO Reports* 2005; **6**, 612–14, www.nature.com/embor/journal/v6/n7/full/7400476.html [accessed 16 January 2014].

26. Disease mongering and drug marketing. 2012. www.drugwatch.com/2012/01/22/disease-mongering-and-drug-marketing [accessed 13 March 2014].

27. Disease mongering debate: creating diseases to sell drugs? 2007. www.familydoctormag.com/medications/118-disease-mongering-debate.html [accessed 13 March 2014].

28. Toon. *Towards a Philosophy of General Practice* (*op. cit.*).

29. Baldwin Research Institute. Alcoholism is not a disease. 2006. www.addictioninfo.org/articles/447/1/Alcoholism-is-not-a-Disease/Page1.html [accessed 16 January 2014].

30. Joint Committee of the American Bar Association and the American Medical Association on Narcotic Drugs. *Drug Addiction, Crime or Disease? Interim and final reports*. Indiana University Press, Library of Congress, www.druglibrary.org/schaffer/library/studies/dacd/default.htm [accessed 16 January 2014].

31. Drug addiction is an illness, not a crime. 2002. www.drug-addiction.com/addiction_is_illness.htm [accessed 16 January 2014].

32. Kaminer W. Is Clinton a sex addict? *Slate*, 22 March 1998, www.slate.com/articles/briefing/articles/1998/03/is_clinton_a_sex_addict.html [accessed 9 May 2014].

33. Thompson S. Is President Clinton a sociopath? *The Ethical Spectacle*, November 1998, www.spectacle.org/1198/righter.html [accessed 16 January 2014].

34. Ellis M. Sex addiction 'not a real disorder'. *Medical News Today*, 22 July 2013, www.medicalnewstoday.com/articles/263750.php [accessed 9 May 2014].

35. When the diagnosis is A.D.H.D. *New York Times*, 15 February 2011, http://consults.blogs.nytimes.com/2011/02/15/when-the-diagnosis-is-a-d-h-d [accessed 16 January 2014].

36. Wolinsky. Disease mongering and drug marketing (*op. cit.*).

37. Kent & Medway PCTs. List of low priority procedures and other procedures with restrictions or thresholds. 2010. Available by request from the Freedom of Information Coordinator at FOI@medway.nhs.uk.

38. Scottish Intercollegiate Guidelines Network. Guideline 117, *Management of Sore Throat and Indications for Tonsillectomy*. Edinburgh: SIGN, 2010. www.sign.ac.uk/pdf/sign117.pdf [accessed 16 January 2014].

39. Harris DL. Cosmetic surgery: where does it begin? *British Journal of Plastic Surgery* 1982; **35**: 281–6.

40. de Sousa A. Concerns about cosmetic surgery. *Indian Journal of Medical Ethics* 2007; **4(4)**: 171–3, http://ijme.in/index.php/ijme/article/view/622/1564 [accessed 1 April 2013].

41. NHS Choices. Get help with prescription costs – medical exemptions. www.nhs.uk/ NHSEngland/Healthcosts/Pages/Prescriptioncosts.aspx [accessed 16 January 2014].

42. NHS Choices. Get help with prescription costs. www.nhs.uk/NHSEngland/Healthcosts/ Pages/Prescriptioncosts.aspx [accessed 16 January 2014].

43. *British National Formulary* § 7.4.5, p. 529 (edition of September 2012).

44. Public Health England. Imported malaria cases and deaths, United Kingdom: 1993–2012. 2013. www.hpa.org.uk/web/HPAweb&HPAwebStandard/HPAweb_C/1195733773780 [accessed 16 January 2014].

45. Cooke FJ, Day M, Wain J, *et al.* Cases of typhoid fever imported into England, Scotland and Wales 2000–2003. *Transactions of the Royal Society of Tropical Medicine and Hygiene* 2007; **101(4)**: 398–404. Epub 2 October 2006.

46. Rull G. Cholera vaccination. 2012. www.patient.co.uk/doctor/Cholera-Vaccination.htm [accessed 16 January 2014].

47. McLeod S. Maslow's Hierarchy of Needs. *Simply Psychology* 2007, updated 2012. www.simplypsychology.org/maslow.html [accessed 16 January 2014].

48. St Paul's Letter to the Ephesians 4: 13.

Chapter 5

Flourishing professionals

In the last two chapters we have glimpsed some of the implications of seeing health care as a MacIntyrean practice in which professionals and patients cooperate to produce the 'internal goods' of health for patients. This view affects our understanding of health and disease, of the purpose of health care and its contribution to health and flourishing. Health is seen not in terms of maximising the quality-adjusted life years (QALYs) of a formless period of time, or conformity to some statistical, social or platonic norm, but as a key element in a life that however long or short has a structure, a purpose and which ends in a good death. An illness is a challenge that is most successfully overcome by the techniques of health care. In so far as it cannot be overcome, the role of health care is to help patients develop an interpretation that helps them to flourish despite the limitations the illness imposes on them. Subjective changes in our expectations of our bodies and minds, and in how we interpret our experiences, are just as important for making our life a story of flourishing as objective changes produced by medical intervention.

MacIntyre's vision therefore does seem to make a difference to health care from the patient's perspective. But what of those who participate as professionals, those for whom health and illness are not intermittently matters of deep personal concern and sometimes literally of life and death, but a daily preoccupation and occupation – the means whereby they earn their living?

The internal goods of health care for professionals

MacIntyre sees taking part in a practice, even if done professionally, not just as an unpleasant activity one puts up with to pay the mortgage but an aspect of life that generates 'internal goods' that make us flourish and make life worth living. In Schumacher's words it is 'good work':[1] an element of our life that contributes to achieving the fullness of our humanity. If this also apply to healthcare professionals then this may answer the question raised in Chapter 1 concerning 'Duties of a doctor'[2] of why health professionals should undertake the difficulties, challenges, and sometimes exacting responsibilities of their profession when they could earn their living more easily in some other way. The flourishing professional engages in the practice not principally for its financial rewards ('external goods'), though these are both necessary and welcome, but for the internal goods they gain from the practice. These goods resemble but go some way beyond the conventional concept of 'job satisfaction'. They vary in detail for different professions within health care, but for most they include the intellectual fascination of the complex problems professionals face, the satisfaction of exercising a high level of skill in addressing those problems, and the personal relationships formed as they do so.

For many doctors it is not hard to see and value these internal goods. Writers such as Heath,[3] Balint,[4] Neighbour[5] and many others have written far more eloquently than I can about how general practice, with its constant variety of problems and privileged access to the lives of people of all ages and types, offers the possibility of being 'A Fortunate Man'[6] or woman. Most healthcare professionals appear to find a continuing interest in what they do, and for few of them does it involve the mind-numbing tedium faced by the filing clerk, the call-centre operator or the factory assembly line worker. Unfortunately there is good evidence that other doctors do not feel this sort of satisfaction from their practice but suffer from 'burnout'.[7] The factors that contribute to burnout are complex,[8] but many of the causes identified can be seen as the result of a distortion of the practice of health care in a morally fragmented society. Under legalistic, managerial and consumerist frameworks professionals are assumed to be driven entirely by external goods and controlled by external forces: rewards, punishments, laws and managerial frameworks. Internal goods are not valued and cultivated.

These external pressures do little to encourage the cultivation of the virtues needed to gain the internal goods. In so far as targets and incentives work they do so by rewarding professionals with 'external goods', usually financial. Rewards rooted in managerialism, even if (like censure and praise) they are not material or limited in quantity, derive much of their power from their scarcity value – they only work if some people don't have them. They are also external to the practice, being contingently rather than intrinsically related to it. If institutional structures and educational processes focus on these external mechanisms to achieve excellence in practice, rather than looking for it to emerge from the internal excellences of practitioners, then the practice is deformed.

As I pointed out in Chapter 1 forces such as managerialism, legalism and consumerism are not only applied to clinicians by managers, lawyers and consumer rights advocates. As well as being taken up by politicians, the media and elements of the general public they are internalised by professionals and become part of their unconscious assumptions. Moral fragmentation becomes not only a feature of society but also part of the individual's psychic structure. The attempt to meet conflicting and incommensurable demands in a morally fragmented practice tends to tear professionals apart as they are pulled in different directions: trying both to maximise health gain and satisfy patients/customers, to do their duty to the person in front of them and respect their rights whilst at the same time using healthcare resources for the greatest good of the greatest number.

As a result it can be hard for practitioners to cultivate the virtues they need to flourish as a professional in the practice. MacIntyre describes[9] how it is impossible to participate fully in a practice and obtain its internal goods if it is seen merely as an end to external goods. Also a practice is a collaborative activity, but as we saw in Chapter 1 many of the moral fragments that currently influence health care encourage competition and adversarial relationships that inhibit collaboration and mutual support.

This does not mean that, even for the flourishing professional, life is or should be one long holiday. There is much satisfaction to be gained from participation in health care as a clinician or manager, and a diagnostic or therapeutic success or the joy that can come from relationships with colleagues and patients could even be described as pleasure. But if one were looking for a life of pleasure then health care would not be the obvious choice, because it brings practitioners close to physical and mental suffering and to death, which is not easy, and requires them to struggle with complex and often intractable problems.

But as Aristotle[10] told us so many centuries ago, a life spent seeking pleasure is not the life worth living. Just as illness is a challenge for patients, achieving the internal goods of health care as a professional is challenging. But as with climbing Everest or crossing the Atlantic singlehanded the challenge is part of the attraction, and one of the features that distinguishes a practice from a pastime. Nussbaum and Sen pointed out that the virtues are the qualities we need to overcome challenges,[11] but it is also through facing the challenges of their role in the practice of health care that professionals develop the virtues needed to gain the internal goods and thereby to flourish.

Challenge is stressful and psychological research and theory makes clear[12] that if stress is to stimulate and not impair performance it needs to be moderated – the Yerkes–Dodson principle.[13] Insufficient challenge fails to provide adequate stimulation and leads to boredom, which may be one cause of burnout – seeing too many sore throats without a narrative that makes them interesting. Conversely, continually facing insoluble problems may be overwhelming and lead to breakdown in performance. Professionals must be equipped with the virtues they need to face the challenges of their professional role, which has important implications for professional education and training.

But this is not only a question of individual personal qualities. The way we organise health care is also important. Practices are collaborative activities, and the support of other practitioners – both fellow professionals and patients – is essential if professionals are to face the challenges of their work and overcome them, growing in virtue. The Balint movement did this for many GPs in the 1950s, by giving them tools to deal with what for them were 'heartsink patients'. It did this partly by providing peer support for isolated practitioners (a trouble shared is a trouble halved) but it also helped doctors find ways to work with the patient to overcome their challenge, moving from an adversarial to a collaborative relationship, and to see not a heartsink patient but an interesting person.

We will consider the implications of this view for the organisation of health care and education and training in Chapter 7. But if this approach to professional practice is to be of practical use we first need to understand what personal qualities or virtues professionals need. These issues have most often been discussed in terms of professionalism in recent years; this discussion of the concept of professionalism provides a good starting point for an account of the virtues the healthcare professional needs to overcome the challenges of practice and so to flourish. We will find in this discussion many of the answers, but we will also see that the concept of professionalism itself has been affected by moral fragmentation and would be strengthened if understood within the framework of health care as a MacIntyrean practice.

Professionalism in a fragmented moral world

There is now a significant literature arising from a concern that professionalism is under threat. A comprehensive review of this literature would be a book in its own right. Many of the key issues were raised in two seminal papers published by the King's Fund[14] and the Royal College of Physicians[15] a decade ago, and they have shaped the discussion that has followed. They make similar points, and the two organisations have subsequently cooperated in exploring the issues further.[16] The King's Fund's *On Being a Doctor* defines professionalism as:

- a calling or vocation linked to public service and altruistic behaviour

- the observance of explicit standards and ethical codes

- the ability to apply a body of specialist knowledge and skills

- a high degree of self-regulation over professional membership and the content and organisation of work.[17]

Both papers identify many of the problems facing health care discussed in Chapter 1 in terms of consumerism, managerialism and legalism as part of the problem with professionalism, although they see them in terms of social change rather than moral fragmentation. For example they speak of:

- an 'increasing expectation among the general public for timely and convenient access to an ever-wider range of services'[18] and a consumerist ethos[19]

- increased managerial control over medical work[20] such as the impact of waiting time initiatives on clinical priorities[21]

- changes in doctors' working conditions that have taken place, driven partly by European legislation restricting working hours[22]

- regulation being offered as the solution to problems with professionalism.[23]

On Being a Doctor speaks of 'the unprecedented challenges arising from the changing expectations of patients, government and managers'.[24]

A more recent review paper from the Health Foundation[25] identifies similar challenges to medical professionalism: social changes that make paternalism unacceptable, coupled with an increased demand to doctors to consider the community perspective and thus sometimes say no to their individual patient ('the new paternalism'); increased regulation and managerial control of doctors; and increase in the need for teamwork alongside a breakdown in trust both between professionals and between professionals and society.

Traditional professionalism?

These publications and others see the changes they identify as eroding 'traditional professionalism':

the traditional image of what this means in practice – a selfless clinician, motivated by a strong ethos of service, equipped with unique skills and knowledge, in control of their work and practising all hours to restore full health to 'his' or 'her' patients.[26]

This may be a nostalgic rose-coloured image of a lost golden age (*O tempora, O mores!*). Certainly George Bernard Shaw did not see physicians in 1911 as selfless clinicians motivated by a strong ethos of service, equipped with unique skills and knowledge, in control of their work and practising all hours to restore full health to their patients. He thought they were 'a conspiracy against the laity'.[27] Even if they were not, few would wish to see a return to practice that is doctor-centred rather than patient-centred, or the haphazard self-regulation by the General Medical Council (GMC) and other professional bodies which eroded the trust that is an essential basis of professionalism.[28]

Recent changes towards partnership between clinician and patient, and the inclusion in regulatory bodies of a wider range of those involved in health care including patients, are a move towards the type of practice outlined in Chapter 2, in which both patients and a variety of professionals have a role to play. Indeed a move towards such a practice may well involve further change in this direction, because sometimes at present patients have token involvement rather than genuine partnership – ticking the 'patient participation' box in the managerialist tool kit. The move from the concept of medical professionalism to 'professionalism in modern health care' – for which the Health Foundation argues – is also in line with this vision of health care. The legalism and managerialism that have come with a more effective, open and democratic system of governance are less helpful, but these are not an inevitable part of these changes.

Philosophical underpinning of the concept of professionalism

Despite professionalism being essentially a moral concept, discussions are seldom grounded in an explicit and philosophically coherent ethical theory; professionalism too floats within the fragments of the moral shipwreck. 'Typically it is seen as combination of values, knowledge and skill, integrity and good judgement in an individual ... other key concepts include character, vocation autonomy and self-regulation'; this is how the Health Foundation[29] report summarises current understanding of medical professionalism. This review also points out that though there have been many attempts to define medical professionalism these have produced little increase in clarity.

Generally the language used of professionalism seems to assume a deontological form of social contract theory, often tinged with values from consumerism, managerialism and legalism. Most authors talk of the duties of doctors; indeed, given the emphasis the GMC places on its document with this title as the bedrock of professionalism, it is hard to avoid doing so. Thus for example the King's Fund says that the first duty of a doctor must be to ensure the wellbeing of patients and to protect them from harm, and puts this responsibility at the heart of medical professionalism.

I pointed out in Chapter 1 that it is hard to see what is in it for doctors in a deontological approach. A social contract framed in terms of external goods – typically power, respect, safety and a good income – is one solution to this difficulty. The social contract is a philosophical fiction that first appeared in the seventeenth century, through which 'imaginary individuals … come together to form a society, accepting obligations of some minimal kind to one another and immediately or very soon after binding themselves to a political sovereign who can enforce those obligations'.[30] The best-known application of the concept in recent times is Rawls's *A Theory of Justice*,[31] in which he considers what people might decide was fair in an 'original position' where the rules of justice are worked out by individuals with no knowledge of what their personal situation is going to be (under the 'veil of ignorance').

The social contract in health care seems to be that professionals make some rather onerous undertakings to provide a good service and not watch the clock; and are given power, prestige and money in return. As with any contract, both parties are in it for what they can get out of it. Since it is framed in terms of external goods it is a zero-sum game, so unless the needs of both parties are perfectly balanced, one or other will feel exploited. One interpretation of the 'crisis in professionalism' is that it is the result of a shift in this balance from one which favoured professionals to one favouring patients.

All the reports mentioned above and many others however speak of professionalism not in terms of a contract but as a 'compact'[32] or an 'implicit compact'.[33] This term implies something similar to a contract but rather less formal, perhaps also including some of the moral undertones of the theological notion of 'covenant',[34] an idea that is important in the Protestant thinking out of which social contract theory evolved.

Another moral fragment sometimes used is the idea of 'vocation'.[35] This originates within a framework of religious belief in which people are 'called' (Latin *vocare*) by God to fulfil a particular role that for them is the best way in which they can 'praise, reverence and serve God and thereby save their souls'.[36]

Although few people see the world in these terms today, certain roles, particularly medicine and nursing, are still sometimes referred to as vocations, although outside the religious tradition in which it originated this concept makes little sense. It is hard to see who is doing the calling, and it can easily become merely an excuse for people to be 'put upon' – we don't need to pay you the going rate because you have a vocation.

How these ideas of duty, the compact and vocation fit together is not clear. Often significant contributions to the discussion of professionalism are philosophically muddled; for example, *On Being a Doctor* suggests that 'The compact must also reflect a duty among doctors to engage in improving health services with a reciprocal obligation on the part of government and managers to develop and implement health policy that allows the highest standards of professional practice to flourish.' How does a compact reflect a duty? And what sense does it make to trade duties for reciprocal obligations? The way out of this muddle is surely to find a coherent moral framework within which the relationship between professionals and patients can be changed from 'zero sum' to 'win-win'. Does MacIntyre's vision offer such an escape route?

A MacIntyrean account of professionalism

An alternative to the philosophical myth of individuals forming a social contract is the image of society as 'the body politic'. The metaphor of society as a body is used by writers as diverse as Aristotle[37] and St Paul,[38] and therefore unsurprisingly by Aquinas whose thinking draws on both these writers. Although this image is not used explicitly by MacIntyre, his vision of flourishing through cooperative practices is clearly rooted in this tradition. The image of society as held together like a body rather than by a contract is a more humane model, emphasising relationships, collaboration, reciprocal roles and mutual benefits. This image fits well with the MacIntyrean vision of health care as a practice outlined in Chapter 2.

Seeing professionalism in terms of virtues, internal goods, flourishing and practices is not an alternative to other visions of professionalism; rather it provides a framework and a rationale for many of the insights of recent discussions of professionalism. For example, accounts of medical professionalism frequently suggest that the 'compact' should include patients and managers as well as doctors; this is in line with the vision of health care as a practice that incorporates patients, managers and clinicians each playing their particular role, as outlined in Chapter 2.

If health care is a practice in this sense, then professionalism is the sum total of the virtues which a professional in that practice needs to gain the internal goods of the practice and to flourish as a professional in that practice. Although discussions of professionalism are usually framed in deontological terms, many of the values seen as crucial in these discussions are actually traditionally virtues:

terms such as integrity and altruism are widely used. Accounts of professionalism frequently speak of professional competence and sound clinical judgement, technical competence and wisdom.[39] It is suggested that doctors should be technically competent, open and honest.[40] Few would dispute this, and these qualities are all aspects of *phronesis* (practical wisdom) – the cardinal virtue that is both moral and intellectual.[41]

Whilst the debate on professionalism does include rudiments of an account of professional virtue, this is from the perspective of character deontology rather than virtue ethics. As in other character deontological accounts, there is no explanation as to why a professional should wish to cultivate these personal qualities. There is no associated account of professional flourishing, or of how the personal qualities professionals need help them overcome the challenges they face in order to flourish. *On Being a Doctor* does speak of professionalism 'flourishing' but not of professionals flourishing or professionalism as flourishing.

An account of professionalism centred on the virtues may lead us to consider qualities less often discussed in recent accounts, such as temperance and self-control, justice and courage. It opens up a vocabulary and a rich literature to help us understand qualities that are important for healthcare professionals but which our society finds hard to discuss, such as humility, love and honour, and it gives us a better perspective than the concept of 'work–life balance' to consider how for professionals the practice of health care fits within their overall life narrative.

Trustworthy professionals

Perhaps the strongest way this vision of professionalism supports other accounts is that the virtues provide a basis for trust. It is generally agreed that trust is the bedrock of professionalism.[42] Patients have to trust their doctors if they are to have confidence in them. O'Neil has recently argued that trustworthiness is prior to trust[43] – a view that implies the sovereignty of virtue. We can only trust someone whom we believe to be virtuous, as Aquinas put it 'to have the habit of acting rightly according to reason' to be trustworthy. This involves believing that they have both the intellectual and the moral virtues to practise adequately – that they are trustworthy. The intellectual virtues include an understanding of the general facts in their area of practice (its evidence base) and the right judgement to apply these facts thoughtfully and appropriately to the situations brought for their attention. Equally they must have the moral virtues discussed above; for example, patients must be able to trust them to be just in their allocation of resources, not distorting their judgement for favouritism or self-interest, temperate in not exploiting their access to their minds and bodies. And so forth.

As *On Being a Doctor* comments, most patients trust doctors whom they know personally. Because it is always easier to trust those whom we know, a practice in need of building trust must make it easier for relationships to grow. This implies if we are to rebuild trust that the present trend driven by consumerism and managerialism away from continuity of care needs to be reversed. But patients also need to be able to approach doctors whom they do not know in the faith that they can trust them. External regulation and incentives alone cannot provide a basis for trust, although if we feel able to trust those who do the regulation to design and implement just systems honestly and with courage they will help. But building a trustworthy profession requires a commitment of the profession as a whole to the internal goods of the practice of health and the virtues needed to achieve those goods with integrity. It also requires both patients and professionals to abandon those fragments of the moral shipwreck that destroy trust – particularly consumerism, legalism, capitalism and perhaps consequentialism.

For the practice to flourish, doctors have to be able to trust their patients too. Patients who conceal pertinent facts from their doctors, or who come with deliberately hidden agendas, will not get the best from their consultations. And patients who approach their doctors from a consumerist or legalist perspective will harm professionalism, whilst those who seek to cultivate the virtues of justice, patience and temperance will contribute to it in a truly collaborative practice.

Trust requires both virtuous professionals and institutions that support the cultivation of those virtues. We will consider what these might look like in the next two chapters.

Notes

1. Schumacher EF. *Good Work*. London: Jonathan Cape, 1979.

2. General Medical Council. Duties of a doctor: the duties of a doctor registered with the General Medical Council. In: *Good Medical Practice*. London: GMC, 2013, www.gmc-uk.org/guidance/good_medical_practice/duties_of_a_doctor.asp [accessed 16 January 2013].

3. Heath I. *The Mystery of General Practice*. London: Nuffield Provincial Hospitals Trust, 1995, www.nuffieldtrust.org.uk/sites/files/nuffield/publication/The_Mystery_of_General_Practice.pdf [accessed 16 January 2013].

4. Balint M. *The Doctor, His Patient and the Illness* (2nd edn). London: Churchill Livingstone, 1964 [1957]. A number of subsequent works published by members of the Balint Society explore the theme further.

5. Neighbour R. *The Inner Consultation*. Dordrecht, Netherlands: Kluwer Academic Publishers Group, 1987.

6. Berger J. *A Fortunate Man: the story of a country doctor*. London: RCGP, 2005.

7. Willacy H. Burnout in the medical profession. 2010. www.patient.co.uk/doctor/burnout-in-the-medical-profession [accessed 16 January 2013].

8. Mayo Clinic Staff. Job burnout: how to spot it and take action. 2012. www.mayoclinic.com/health/burnout/WL00062 [accessed 16 January 2013].

9. MacIntyre A. *After Virtue: a study in moral theory* (2nd edn). London: Duckworth, 1985.

10. Aristotle. *The Ethics of Aristotle: the Nicomachean ethics* (trans. JAK Thomson). Harmondsworth: Penguin, 1955, Book X § i–iv.

11. Nussbaum MC, Sen A. *The Quality of Life*. Oxford: Clarendon Press, 1993.

12. Sincero SM. How does stress affect performance? 2012. http://explorable.com/how-does-stress-affect-performance [accessed 16 January 2013].

13. Cherry K. What is the Yerkes–Dodson Law? http://psychology.about.com/od/yindex/f/yerkes-dodson-law.htm [accessed 16 January 2013].

14. Rosen R, Dewar S. *On Being a Doctor: redefining medical professionalism for better patient care*. London: King's Fund, 2004, www.kingsfund.org.uk/publications/being-doctor-medical-professionalism [accessed 16 January 2013].

15. Royal College of Physicians. *Doctors in Society: medical professionalism in a changing world*. Report of a working party. London: RCP, 2005, www.rcplondon.ac.uk/sites/default/files/documents/doctors_in_society_reportweb.pdf [accessed 16 January 2013].

16. Levenson R, Dewar S, Shepherd S. *Understanding Doctors: harnessing professionalism*. London: King's Fund, 2008, www.kingsfund.org.uk/publications/understanding-doctors [accessed 16 January 2013].

17. Rosen, Dewar. *On Being a Doctor (op. cit.)*.

18. Rosen, Dewar. *On Being a Doctor (op. cit.)*.

19. Royal College of Physicians. *Doctors in Society (op. cit.)*.

20. Rosen, Dewar. *On Being a Doctor (op. cit.)*.

21. Royal College of Physicians. *Doctors in Society (op. cit.)*.

22. Rosen, Dewar. *On Being a Doctor (op. cit.)*.

23. Royal College of Physicians. *Doctors in Society (op. cit.)*.

24. Rosen, Dewar. *On Being a Doctor (op. cit.)*.

25. Christmas S, Millward L. *New Medical Professionalism*. A scoping report for the Health Foundation. London: Health Foundation, 2011, www.health.org.uk/public/cms/75/76/313/2733/New%20medical%20professionalism.pdf?realName=JOGEKF.pdf accessed [accessed 16 January 2013].

26. Rosen, Dewar. *On Being a Doctor (op. cit.)*.

27. Shaw GB. *The Doctor's Dilemma*. London: Constable & Co., 1935 [1911] and many other editions. First performed 1911.

28. Koehn D. *The Ground of Professional Ethics*. London: Routledge, 1994

29. Christmas, Millward. *New Medical Professionalism (op. cit.)*.

30. Honderich T. Social contract. In: *Oxford Companion to Philosophy*. Oxford: Oxford University Press, 1995, pp. 163–4.

31. Rawls J. *A Theory of Justice*. Oxford: Oxford University Press, 1972.

32. Christmas, Millward. *New Medical Professionalism (op. cit.)*.

33. Rosen, Dewar. *On Being a Doctor (op. cit.)*.

34. Westminster Confession of Faith. 1646. Chapter VII – Of God's covenant with man. www.reformed.org/documents/wcf_with_proofs [accessed 16 January 2013].

35. Christmas, Millward. *New Medical Professionalism (op. cit.)*.

36. Ignatius of Loyola. *First Principle and Foundation – spiritual exercises*. Christian Ethereal Classics. www.ccel.org/ccel/ignatius/exercises.xii.i.html [accessed 16 January 2013].

37. Aristotle. *Politics*. Trans. TA Sinclair 1962, rev. TJ Saunders. Harmondsworth: Penguin, 1981.

38. St Paul. First Epistle to the Corinthians 12.

39. Royal College of Physicians. *Doctors in Society (op. cit.)*.

40. Rosen, Dewar. *On Being a Doctor (op. cit.)*.

41. Aristotle. *Ethics (op. cit.)*.

42. Koehn. *The Ground of Professional Ethics (op. cit.)*.

43. O'Neil O. *A Point of View: which comes first – trust or trustworthiness?* Radio talk, 7 December 2012, www.bbc.co.uk/podcasts/series/pov/all. Transcript at www.bbc.co.uk/news/magazine-20627410 [accessed 16 January 2013].

Chapter 6

Some thoughts on professional virtue

A full account of professional virtue and flourishing professional narratives would be the work of a lifetime. Moreover, the standards of excellence of a practice cannot be defined by one person; they are the product of a tradition to which all practitioners contribute. In health care this must include patients, managers and other health professionals as well as doctors – the Health Foundation's 'new medical professionalism'.[1] And perhaps these virtues can only be fully understood as they are lived rather than from general accounts of them; we need 'narrative ethics'. A few thoughts on some of the virtues medical professionals require may however give some ideas of what such an account might look like and how we might set about developing it.

The bulk of this chapter will be devoted to a consideration of compassion and how it relates to flourishing, but I will also include some thoughts on other virtues that do not always get the attention they deserve, particularly temperance and the very Aristotelian concept of honour or magnanimity, and how all these virtues relate to professional altruism.

Compassion and flourishing

An important theme of the Francis Report[2] and other recent discussions of problems in the health service is that professionals need to be more compassionate. But it is not always clear what we mean by compassion, or how this fits with the central axiom of virtue ethics that possessing and exercising the virtues, including compassion, is the best route to a flourishing life. Can compassion and flourishing coexist, or is the call for greater compassion merely adding another burden to already overloaded professionals?

What is flourishing?

First of all we must remember, as discussed in Chapter 2, that flourishing is not the same as continuous pleasure or a feeling of wellbeing. Just as a plant often flourishes better if it is pruned, so a human being may ultimately have a fuller life if it includes coping with setbacks and periods of suffering. Life has an element of tragedy in it, and unpleasant feelings are an important part of life as much as pleasant ones. Suffering and joy are both part of the human condition and our world view is diminished and our humanity stunted if we don't allow ourselves to experience that. A person with dulled sensations, walled off from his feelings, is not living a fully human life. If we cut ourselves off from negative emotions we risk also cutting ourselves off from those which give us great joy. As HRH Queen Elizabeth II quoted after the 9/11 attacks, 'the pain of grief is the price we pay for love.'[3]

Flourishing means having a rich life – loving, delighting in beauty and learning about the awesome, complex world in which we find ourselves. But it will also involve suffering, loss and death, which (with it is said taxes) are part of human life we all share. For almost all of us flourishing involves relationships that carry the risk of loss and grief. If we are to survive and flourish in our wonderful but rather frightening world we need the virtues, the personal qualities that allow us to deal with challenges successfully in a way that enhances rather than diminishes our humanity.

Because life involves illness and death sooner or later, these are challenges all of us have to face personally, but those who work in health care, whether as clinicians, administrators or managers, will certainly also have to face them professionally time and time again. How can professionals cope with that with compassion?

Limits to professional suffering

Literally compassion means 'suffering with' from the Latin *com*, with and *passum*, the participle of the deponent verb *patior*, I suffer, from which we also get patient, patience, passion and passive. In general usage however the term has shifted a little from a focus on shared suffering. Two different dictionaries give very similar definitions: 'Deep awareness of the suffering of another coupled with the wish to relieve it'[4] and 'a feeling of deep sympathy and sorrow for another who is stricken by misfortune, accompanied by a strong desire to alleviate the suffering'[5]. Both definitions have two parts: an awareness or feeling aroused by suffering or misfortune, and a desire to alleviate it.

The first part of these definitions gives us a clue as to why people might think compassion and flourishing are incompatible for health professionals: the arousal of feeling by suffering. In his blog on the placebo effect Daniel Jacobs comments that:

> *Throughout much of the history of western medicine, it was believed that a doctor's role in a doctor-patient relationship was to detach from the emotional needs of a patient, listen to the maladies, make a diagnosis if needed, and prescribe a solution. Providing emotional support was believed to make a diagnosis harder, as it hindered doctors in making an objective assessment of the patient's situation.*[6]

I don't know how true Jacobs's historical generalisation is, but medical teachers often suggest that as medical students become better at objective assessments of patients, their awareness of what it feels like to be the patient diminishes, and there is some evidence to support this.[7]

Attachment and detachment

The intellectual activity of turning a patient's story into a diagnosis that clarifies possible courses of action does require a certain emotional detachment. If clinicians get too upset they can't think clearly, and understanding the patient's problems in terms of pathology and pathophysiology means viewing their bodies as objects – an *I-it* rather than an *I-Thou* relationship, to use Buber's terminology.[8] Also, sometimes clinicians have to do things that cause pain or discomfort to patients – if they were too frightened of hurting someone to elicit tenderness on abdominal palpation, to give injections or take blood they couldn't do their job.

In fact health care also requires a degree of emotional detachment from their suffering in patients, too. A few patients see the consultation as the opportunity for a good moan, or a chance to convince the doctor how bad their pain is. This excessive emphasis on the emotional rather than the factual element of their symptoms can sometimes get in the way of solving their problems.

One way clinicians deal with the need for emotional detachment is to try to stop feeling – to become callous, to grow a hard shell around them so that they cease to feel their patient's suffering. This is understandable, because as T.S. Eliot put it 'humankind cannot bear too much reality'.[9] Clinicians couldn't function if they felt the full horror of some of the suffering they encounter; it would destroy them. But there is evidence throughout history that those who allow themselves to witness but not be aware of the suffering of others run terrible risks. This degree of emotional detachment from the feelings of others can enable people to inflict the sort of torture and ill-treatment seen all too often in people seeking asylum, and in extreme cases to the inhumanity seen in the concentration camps of the Nazi Holocaust.[10] In less extreme cases but closer to home it leads to the events at Mid Staffordshire Hospital described in the Francis Report.[11] This jeopardises our flourishing both as professionals and as human beings.

The value of feelings

Also, as the Balint movement has demonstrated,[12] feeling the patient's emotions is an important diagnostic tool for clinicians. Much of the power of the Balint group lies in how it sensitises us to the emotional responses patients produce in us, and teaches us to use them positively. Thus a doctor notices a patient makes her angry, and this points her to a diagnosis of depression. A doctor's feeling of helplessness and confusion faced with a patient's story may reflect the patient's confusion and sense of powerlessness faced with an illness. Balint also pointed out that 'the drug doctor'[13] is an important therapeutic tool that relies on emotional awareness and emotional contact in the consultation. This is an important element in what Jacobs and many others call the placebo effect.

Awareness of their own emotions by clinicians also stops them getting in the way; for example when one notices that a patient who is irritating for no obvious reason reminds us of an elderly relative we can't stand. And psychoanalysis shows us that emotions that are suppressed or repressed sometimes manifest themselves in other much nastier ways. So feelings can be useful aids or dangerous obstacles to clinicians in their work. Clinicians can't function properly if they ignore them or try to abolish them, so they have to find ways to deal with them.

Managing our feelings

In *The Inner Consultation*[14] the GP teacher Roger Neighbour suggested it is helpful to think of the encounter between doctor and patient in terms of 'two heads'. One, which he calls the Organiser, is the intellectual part of the brain, analysing and planning, thinking logically and being in control. The other he calls the Responder – intuitive, picking up verbal and non-verbal cues, noticing patterns and being aware of the doctor's emotional responses. This idea is helpful in understanding what goes on in a healthcare consultation, but perhaps we can 'unpack' the second head, the Responder, and using the traditional image of the seat of the emotions, think of having two heads and a heart. Our emotional response to the situation, what our heart is telling us, is important data for our Responder head; that head also needs to keep track of where our heart is taking us, so that it doesn't push us off the rails.

Neighbour also talks about 'housekeeping' – the habit clinicians need to develop of clearing both their mind and their heart at the end of one consultation so as to be ready to move on to the next. This is an important part of dealing with our emotional responses to the suffering of patients without blocking them out completely. One point he makes as part of his discussion of how to do this is the importance of being in the here and now: the habit of being very aware of the feelings of the patient when we are with them. This is in part the importance of 'being there' emphasised by Paul Julian[15] – perhaps something that is increasingly difficult as in general we get used to moving through the world in our own 'bubble' created by iPods and mobile phones, and in the consultation the computer brings the wider agenda of health care to our desktops. But being there also involves letting go of our feelings and our involvement with the patient once we have parted – being in the present of the new situation. This is perhaps one of the keys to flourishing as a clinician who can have feelings aroused by the suffering of others but not be overwhelmed by them.

The desire to alleviate suffering

So reflecting on the definition of compassion as involving awareness of suffering seems to help us understand how the emotions aroused by suffering can be compatible with flourishing. Although the second part of the definitions also suggest emotion in speaking of desire to alleviate suffering, desire here perhaps means primarily motivation rather than emotion, although like all strong motivations this desire is not devoid of feeling. If desire to alleviate suffering is not the motivation of health care, and of all health professionals, it is hard to see what the health service is for. Even the bureaucratic NHS Constitution acknowledges that:

> The NHS is there to improve our health and wellbeing, supporting us to keep mentally and physically well, to get better when we are ill and, when we cannot fully recover, to stay as well as we can to the end of our lives.[16]

I do however remember once being rendered speechless when trying to admit an old lady, living on her own, who had gone 'off her legs'. After I'd explained that I could find no obvious reason why she had become unable to get about and care for herself the registrar said, 'So you are just asking me to admit her for compassionate reasons, then?' What other reason could there be for an admission to hospital other than a desire to alleviate the patient's suffering, coupled with a hope that this would help? Emotions aren't just slushy feelings we wallow in – they are essential motivators to action. And this is another reason why we should not, indeed dare not, learn not to feel: if we don't feel anything for the suffering of patients then we will at best become indifferent to their suffering and at worst become able to be cruel as torturers and concentration camp guards can be cruel.

So thinking about the derivation and meaning of compassion helps us understand why it's important to flourishing. Compassion is a natural response to suffering that motivates what we do as clinicians. It damages our humanity and our clinical expertise if we suppress it, but we need to be able to deal with the emotional element of it effectively.

Synonyms for compassion

Words don't exist in isolation; clusters of words are close in meaning and often overlap. One way to understand the meaning of compassion is to look at words close in meaning to compassion. This might give us some further clues as to how best, most virtuously to cope with the endless stress of human misery that clinicians encounter – some of it major, much of it rather minor – but never minor to the person suffering at the time.

The synonyms for compassion from a modern online thesaurus[17] are:

> benevolence, charity, clemency, commiseration, compunction, condolence, consideration, empathy, fellow feeling, grace, heart, humaneness, humanity, kindness, lenity, mercy, softheartedness, softness, sorrow, sympathy, tenderheartedness, tenderness, yearning

Whilst the classic thesaurus of 1911 by Roget[18] gives:

pity, compassion, commiseration; bowels of compassion; sympathy, fellow-feeling, tenderness, yearning, forbearance, humanity, mercy, clemency; leniency &c. (lenity) ... charity, ruth, long-suffering

(which incidentally shows how our language has changed since 1911 – few people these days use the word *ruth*, although the opposite *ruthless* is still in common use; or use *lenity*, or think of the bowels as the seat of compassion).

Beneficence, one of Beauchamp and Childress's four ethical principles,[19] which are supposed to underlie health care, doesn't appear in either list. Beneficence – doing good (from Latin *bene*, good and *facere*, to do) is however very close to benevolence – wishing good (from Latin *bene*, good and *volere*, to wish), which heads the more modern list. These two words are closely linked in life as well as in etymology. Usually people do good because they wish to do so, although occasionally they may do so by accident, and one may sometimes wish to do good but fail to do so – through ignorance, weakness of will, or for reasons outside your control.

But we rarely speak of benevolence in relation to health care, and perhaps this dog that doesn't bark[20] gives us a second clue as to why people are nervous about talking about compassion in health care. In our patient-centred world that prizes autonomy, benevolence smacks of paternalism, and this is a dirty word. This is not because of the strict meaning of the word but because of how it is commonly used. Victorian industrialists were benevolent if they looked after their staff and didn't exploit them; their wives demonstrated their benevolence by taking soup to the poor and knitting them socks. We are rightly suspicious of the attitudes that underlie these actions today, and hence avoid using the word.

Sympathy and empathy

It is similarly hard to use the word pity, Roget's first synonym for compassion, because its common usage today also suggests someone looking down paternalistically – although again the original meaning and etymology (from Latin *pietas* – piety, duty, loyalty[21]) does not imply this. Sympathy has suffered a similar fate. A blog entry encapsulates this:

I myself find the word Sympathise one of the most patronising words about, more so if a death has occurred. Some people don't want sympathy, just an understanding. I find Empathise a more subtle word.[22]

The belief that empathy is preferable to sympathy because it is not patronising seems quite common. Robin Edmondson however has done a nice piece of work comparing definitions of the two terms.[23] She summarises it thus:

Sympathy: I am sorry for your loss. What can I do to help you during this difficult time?

Empathy: I feel and understand your pain; my grandmother passed away last year as well.

This implies that you can always feel sympathy, but to be empathic you must have had a similar experience to the person who suffers. If clinicians have faced a similar situation to the patient then they can share their feelings empathically, and no doubt this can be useful. But this will often not be the case, and if they try to be empathic by pretending they have – saying 'I know how you feel' when they don't – that is dishonest and may sound false, even condescending. Conversely, genuine sympathy is neither false nor condescending. As a patient I remember having a catheter removed, and the female nurse who did it said something like 'I don't have the same plumbing but I'm sure it must hurt like hell, so swear all you like' – an expression of sympathy that didn't feel at all patronising, but showed humanity.

This analysis of the meaning of the terms suggests that both empathy and sympathy can be patronising or genuine expressions of compassion, in one case entering into the suffering of a person from experience and in the other from imagination. It all depends on how they are felt and expressed.

Suffering alongside

Both empathy and sympathy can involve a degree of suffering with – not the same suffering as the person afflicted, but sometimes as hard to bear. Compassion is an important theme in all the world's religions, but perhaps the most famous image of sympathetic suffering in Western culture is of Mary the Mother of Jesus and St John standing at the foot of Jesus dying on the cross. In the Middle Ages an image of this scene would have been in almost every church in England. Even today most art galleries in Europe contain a representation of it, one of which is shown in Figure 6.1.

A medieval poet inspired by this image poignantly asks:

Quis est homo qui non fleret,

matrem Christi si videret

in tanto supplicio?[24]

[Who would not weep to see a mother in such a situation?]

Clinical compassion is often like this. We don't share the suffering of the patient, but we see it and that involves its own suffering. Obviously we feel less for a patient than we would for a son or a close friend, but if we don't feel sad when we see suffering, be it physical like that of the crucified or mental like that of his mother, we are less than fully human.

Quite often the compassion of clinicians is like that of Mary the Mother of Jesus and St John in another way – all we can do is stand there with the person suffering. That can be valuable – Julian's 'being there' again. But sometimes we can also do something a little more practical. Another common image in Western art is Simon of Cyrene, who was press-ganged into helping Jesus carry his cross. In Chris Gollon's representation of the Stations of the Cross[25] *Simon the Cyrenean Helps Jesus* (see Figure 6.2) shows deep humanity in Simon's face, whilst in *Jesus is Condemned to Death* the faces of the Romans sentencing Jesus to death are distorted and grotesque (see Figure 6.3). This is a powerful illustration of the fact that to be fully human you need compassion.

Figure 6.1: Matthias Grünewald's *Large Crucifixion* (the Tauberbischofsheim Altarpiece), 1523–25

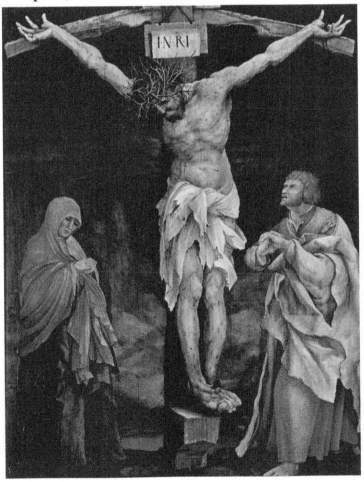

Figure 6.2: Simon the Cyrenean Helps Jesus

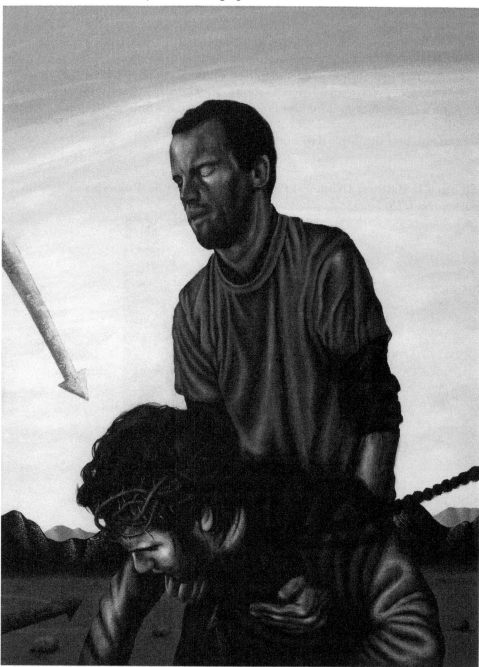

Stations of the Cross (V): Simon the Cyrenean Helps Jesus © Chris Gollon
(www.chrisgollon.com).

Figure 6.3: Jesus is Condemned to Death

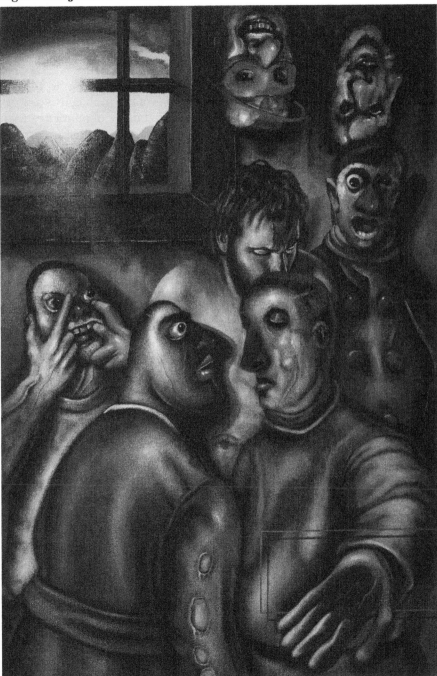

Stations of the Cross (I): Jesus is Condemned to Death © Chris Gollon
(www.chrisgollon.com).

The four loves

Perhaps, however, the most important synonym for compassion on the thesaurus lists is charity. This word comes from the Latin *caritas*, now usually translated into English as love because like benevolence the word charity has become tarnished and is not often used today except to describe organisations. I've not been able to trace the origin of the phrase 'cold as charity' but most people seem to think it relates to the unfeeling, regimented public institutions of the nineteenth century more concerned with keeping budgets down and preventing dependency than helping people in a spirit of love. Perhaps that rings bells about values in some of our public services today!

It sounds a bit odd to say that we should love our patients, but I think a reflection on love might help us understand compassion and flourishing in health care better. In Greek there are four words for love, and C.S. Lewis explored them in some detail.[26] He may have overemphasised the distinction between the four, both in how we experience love and in how people use the words. They overlapped in Ancient Greek, and they overlap in our lives too, but characterising, even caricaturing them, may teach us something about love, compassion and flourishing in the context of health care.

Eros, passionate or erotic love, is usually thought of as the sort of love you fall in, like a bear trap. In Ancient Greece it was seen as a form of madness – perhaps closer to lust than love in modern English usage. Plato argued for a more sophisticated approach to *eros*, from which presumably we get 'the platonic relationship' (although Plato's relationships were far from platonic in the modern sense). Whether platonic or raw in tooth and claw, this type of love has no place in relationships between clinicians and patients, and can lead to uncomfortable conversations with the GMC and other regulatory bodies. But we do need to develop the habit of recognising *eros* when it enters clinician–patient relationships, and taking action to nip it in the bud.

Often it comes from the patient, as an exaggerated transference reaction. This can be very seductive; it is very flattering to be told by patients that they always want to see us, and that because we are so much better than other doctors, we understand their problems as no one else does. This may be perfectly innocent, but when it escalates to telling us how beautiful and special we are, alarm bells need to ring. But *eros* can also come from the clinician. In an anonymous Dutch survey of ENT surgeons and gynaecologists[27] 85% admitted to being sexually attracted to their patients at some time. It's tempting to wonder whether the other 15% had very unattractive patients or were lying! Sexual attraction is part of being human, and just because someone is a patient it doesn't abolish our instinctive response to their sexuality. But it should affect what we do about it, and here the virtue of self-control is crucial. Although we will have feelings about patients, we need to be able to control them – this applies to all our feelings, but the consequences on not controlling feelings of sexual attraction are particularly disastrous. It is worrying that the same survey reported that 4% admitted to having had sexual relations with patients.

Storge means affection – often between family members, but one can imagine how, particularly in a longstanding relationship, it can apply to patients. General practitioners and indeed hospital doctors who have treated patients for many years often speak fondly of them, with a feeling perhaps not that different from how we feel about aunts, uncles and cousins. The main problem with this is that it depends on the personality of the person – there are patients we know just as well and for as long for whom our feelings are better described as irritation and exasperation than affection. As C.S. Lewis points out,[28] this happens in families too! But justice demands that we don't treat patients better because we like them or less favourably because they get on our nerves – or at least that we try not to. This is one reason why justice has to be a virtue as well as a principle.

Philia is friendship – the love Aristotle thought was one of the main things that led to *eudaemonia*. When I explored the boundaries of the ill-defined relationship between GP and patient[29] I suggested that sometimes the GP acts as a concerned friend – which can be virtuous or disastrous, depending on the situation. This type of love shares with *storge* the problem that not all patients elicit it. In any group there are a few with whom we 'click' – we share common interests and find their company agreeable. All doctors find some patients interesting, fun to be with, and easy to empathise with; others are less attractive or are frankly irritating.

But making friends of some of our patients can lead us to be unjust to others. Justice, another core professional virtue, requires that our friendship or lack of it should make no difference to how patients are treated. In some ways this is harder than resisting sexual attraction, because the line between the acceptable and the unacceptable is fuzzier. It is never good practice to grope or seduce your patients, but it is good practice to spend time talking about non-medical matters and to take an interest in them as people, not just as problems. Justice however demands that the clinician does not favour the young, attractive and intelligent over the old, ugly and stupid in this respect.

Conversely, controlling aversion to particular individuals or type of patient is also important and often difficult. A clinician may find particular mannerisms, manners of speech or attitudes and beliefs irritating; or (particularly for the general practitioner working in a small community) she may know that an individual has done things of which she disapproves, and even have other patients or friends who have been harmed by that person. Putting aside our emotional response to such situations is a challenge to the clinician's virtue of self-control.

Self-knowledge, self-control and the unity of the virtues

These discussions of *eros, storge* and *philia* remind us that professionals need to be able to recognise and control desires and other feelings both positive and negative that impair their performance within the practice. Most obviously they must control sexual feelings that patients may arouse in them; this is particularly important for clinicians because their role involves physical contact. If as may well happen a clinician needs to examine a person whom he finds physically attractive, professionalism means never allowing these feelings to make the slightest difference to the clinician's behaviour, and never allowing the patient to be aware of them. The same applies to emotional attraction to patients.

This also illustrates another important concept in virtue ethics: 'the unity of the virtues'. Although we need accounts of individual virtues, they do not exist in isolation. To be compassionate involves self-knowledge and self-control, and without all these (and other qualities that we have not considered such as courage and temperance) one cannot have the virtue of justice. This is another reason why the value of general accounts of virtue such as this is limited; it is only as they work out in particular situations that we see how the virtues link together and reinforce each other.

The fourth love

The last of CS Lewis's loves is *agape* – usually translated into Latin as *caritas* (which originally in Latin meant preciousness, dearness, high price), and into English as charity before the word got tarnished. It means love for people irrespective of their personal qualities and their behaviour.

The best-known definition of this sort of love comes from St Paul in a passage[30] often read both at weddings and funerals. He describes love as patient, kind, not envious or boastful or arrogant or rude, not insisting on its own way, not irritable or resentful; not rejoicing in wrongdoing, but rejoicing in the truth.

This I think is as good a definition of compassion as you can get. And it's also a good part of a definition of the qualities we need to live a flourishing life as we struggle through the choppy waters of health care: patience, kindness, politeness, calmness.

Cultivating these virtues is of course easier said than done. But a curious feature of the translation of *agape* into Latin might give us a final clue as to how we might set about doing that. In Greek *agape* is a noun but it has a cognate verb – *agapao*. Latin however does not have a verb form of *caritas* – you either have to say someone 'has charity' or you use a different verb – *diligo, diligere, dilexi, dilectum*. The main meaning of this verb seems to be to elect, to choose out, and by extension it means to value, to prize and to love. It has a broad range or meanings including care about, like, enjoy, hold dear, esteem, value, have special regard for.[31]

Enjoy is perhaps a particularly interesting meaning. Etymologists suggest the word 'delectation' – to enjoy, to delight in – derives from a medieval Latin verb *delectatio*, but it is so similar to *dilectum*, the past participle of *diligo*, that one can't help wondering whether there is a link. Whether or not this etymological speculation is correct, finding ways to enjoy, to delight in patients, is one thing that helps clinicians go on '*agape*-ing' them and being compassionate to them, and through that enjoyment, that delight, that love, both to show compassion and to flourish.

Temperance as a professional virtue

The importance of temperance in its narrow sense to professionalism is obvious; one only has to see how excessive use of alcohol commonly brings doctors to the attention of the GMC. But other aspects of temperance involving work, rest and fitness are important too if one is to flourish in the demanding role of a professional. There is a longstanding tradition of 'workaholism' in health care that often distorts the practice away from promoting flourishing. Although commitment to work can be fulfilling for professionals, there needs to be a right balance between the practice of health care and other practices – parenthood, tennis, choral singing, or whatever other practices play a significant part in the life of the individual – for a flourishing narrative to be constructed. The mixture will be different for every individual, but failure to find the right balance can be disastrous to both professional life and personal relationships.

Accepting the uncomfortable fact that, however hard we try, we cannot always be able to offer a cure, and will not always get the diagnosis right, whilst continuing to be committed to do our best and strive to be better, is perhaps another aspect of temperance.

Integrity and honour as a barrier against malpractice

The concept of honour has had a bad press recently, because it has been used to justify ill-treatment of those seen as having damaged a family's honour and is associated with 'honour killings'. Like benevolence it also has a rather old-fashioned condescending feeling; being concerned with one's honour was a sign you belonged to the upper classes. But there is a more positive view of honour that may be helpful to us: that a person's self-image will not allow him to act in a way that is wrong or ignoble. The self-image of oneself as a professional will not allow one to act other than professionally. So the virtuous professional will act rightly not because the rules say she must (though 'v-rules' are useful in guiding her in what to do and in strengthening her resolve to do it) nor because there are rewards for good conduct and sanctions for doing wrong (though these too are useful stimuli), but because it is not in her nature to act in any other way. This is what underlies '*noblesse oblige*', an idea that, although rooted in a society far more hierarchical than ours, is relevant to us because illness makes the strongest people vulnerable, however much professionals seek to work in partnership with patients. Therefore not to treat them well would be dishonourable, and like Frederick Douglass the virtuous professional would say 'I prefer to be true to myself, even at the hazard of incurring the ridicule of others, rather than to be false, and to incur my own abhorrence.' Honour is one word for this view of oneself; another is integrity.

Other neglected virtues

These are just some examples of virtues clinicians need to flourish. I discussed the virtues of courage (commonly moral and less often physical), and hope briefly, in *Towards a Philosophy of General Practice.*[32] Other neglected virtues that merit further exploration include patience, discretion (the ability to refrain from speaking) and humility.

Justice is usually thought of as a moral principle, but it is also a virtue, and as the role of GPs increasingly involves the general wellbeing of the community as well as the needs of their individual patients its importance becomes clearer. As with professionalism in general there is much in the existing literature that contributes towards accounts of these virtues, even if not explicitly labelled as such, for example, the RCGP Ethics Committee's guidance on commissioning[33] is an excellent starting point for an account of justice.

Virtue and altruism

Most definitions of professionalism speak of altruism in some way or another. This suggests placing the interests of patients above those of the physician. Thus for example *On Being a Doctor* suggests that professionalism requires that the 'patient's interests are put at the heart of professional practice'. Seen as a duty this is onerous, but seen in terms of the virtue of compassion and the other virtues discussed above it is enlightened self-interest. It is through these virtues, which can be summarised as professional altruism and through commitment to the purpose of the practice and its internal goods for the patient, that professionals obtain their internal goods, which are their chief reward from the practice.

In the practice of the theatre discussed in Chapter 2, the professional obtains those goods to some extent by losing himself in the practice – we often speak of an actor 'giving a performance'. Actors gain enormously from this experience, but they do so by doing it not for themselves but for the audience. In a similar way a MacIntyrean view suggests that, although professional altruism may at times seem costly, it is amply rewarded in terms of internal goods.

Notes

1. Christmas S, Millward L. *New Medical Professionalism*. A scoping report for the Health Foundation. London: Health Foundation, 2011, www.health.org.uk/public/cms/75/76/313/2733/New%20medical%20professionalism.pdf?realName=JOGEKF.pdf accessed [accessed 16 January 2013].

2. Francis R. *Independent Inquiry into Care Provided by Mid Staffordshire NHS Foundation Trust: January 2005–March 2009*. Volume 1. London: The Stationery Office, 2013, http://webarchive.nationalarchives.gov.uk/20130107105354/http://www.dh.gov.uk/prod_consum_dh/groups/dh_digitalassets/@dh/@en/@ps/documents/digitalasset/dh_113447.pdf [accessed 16 January 2014].

3. Sapsted D, Foster P, Jones G. Grief is price of love, says the Queen. *Daily Telegraph*, 21 September 2001, www.telegraph.co.uk/news/worldnews/northamerica/usa/1341155/Grief-is-price-of-love-says-the-Queen.html [accessed 16 January 2014].

4. www.thefreedictionary.com/compassion [accessed 16 January 2014].

5. http://dictionary.reference.com/browse/compassion [accessed 16 January 2014].

6. Jacobs D. A good doctor-patient relationship creates a strong placebo effect. 18 February 2013. www.placeboeffect.com/doctor-patient-relationship [accessed 16 January 2014].

7. Hebert PC, Meslin EM, Dunn EV. Measuring the ethical sensitivity of medical students: a study at the University of Toronto. *Journal of Medical Ethics* 1992; **18(3)**: 142–7.

8. Buber M. *I and Thou* (2nd edn). New York: Macmillan, 1984.

9. Eliot TS. *Burnt Norton* (1936). *Complete Poems and Plays*. London: Faber & Faber, 1972.

10. United States Holocaust Memorial Museum. Introduction to the Holocaust. 2013. www.ushmm.org/wlc/en/article.php?ModuleId=10005143 [accessed 16 January 2014].

11. Francis R. *Independent Inquiry (op. cit.)*.

12. Pennine GP Training Scheme. Briefing for Balint groups. 2009. www.pennine-gp-training.co.uk/balint-groups.doc [accessed 16 January 2014].

13. Balint M. *The Doctor, His Patient and the Illness* (2nd edn). London: Livingstone, 1964 [1957].

14. Neighbour R. *The Inner Consultation*. Dordrecht, Netherlands: Kluwer Academic Publishers Group, 1987.

15. Julian P. Being there. In: A Elder, O Samuel (eds), *While I'm Here, Doctor: a study of the doctor/patient relationship*. London: Tavistock Publications, 1987, pp. 77–83.

16. Department of Health. *The NHS Constitution*. London: DH, 2013, www.nhs.uk/choiceintheNHS/Rightsandpledges/NHSConstitution/Documents/2013/the-nhs-constitution-for-england-2013.pdf [accessed 16 January 2014].

17. http://thesaurus.com/browse/compassion.

18. *Roget's Thesaurus*. London: Everyman, 1991.

19. Beauchamp TL, Childress JF. *Principles of Biomedical Ethics*. New York: Oxford University Press, 1989.

20. Doyle AC. Silver Blaze. In: *The Memoirs of Sherlock Holmes*. 1892. http://en.wikisource.org/wiki/Silver_Blaze [accessed 16 January 2014].

21. www.etymonline.com/index.php?term=pity [accessed 16 January 2014].

22. www.thinkypedia.com/question/13182 [accessed 16 January 2014].

23. Edmonson R. Difference between sympathy and empathy: grammar guide. 2007. http://hubpages.com/hub/Sympathy_vs_Empathy [accessed 16 January 2014].

24. Jacopone da Todi. Stabat Mater Dolorosa. Thirteenth century – also attributed to Pope Innocent III and St Bonaventure. www.preces-latinae.org/thesaurus/BVM/SMDolorosa. html [accessed 16 January 2014].

25. Gollon C. *The Stations of the Cross* – a series of paintings hung in St John's Church, Bethnal Green, London E2 9PA. Photographs of the paintings can be seen at www.chrisgollon. com/collections/stations-of-the-cross [accessed 16 January 2014].

26. Lewis CS. *The Four Loves*. London: Collins, 1960.

27. Wilbers D, Veenstra G, van de Wiel HBM, *et al.* Sexual contact in the doctor-patient relationship in The Netherlands. *British Medical Journal* 1992; **304**: 1531–4.

28. Lewis. *The Four Loves* (*op. cit.*).

29. Toon PD. Setting boundaries: a virtue approach to the clinician-patient relationship in primary care. In: D Bowman, J Spicer (eds), *Primary Care Ethics*. Abingdon: Radcliffe Publishing, 2007, pp. 83–99.

30. St Paul. First Letter to the Corinthians 13.

31. www.latinwordlist.com/latin-words/diligo-8063308.htm [accessed 6 May 2014].

32. Toon PD. *Towards a Philosophy of General Practice* (Occasional Paper 78). London: RCGP, 1998.

33. Oswald M, Cox D. *Making Difficult Choices: ethical commissioning guidance to general practitioners*. London: RCGP, 2011, www.rcgp.org.uk/~/media/Files/News/RCGP-Ethical-Commissioning-Guidance.ashx [accessed 16 January 2014].

Chapter 7

Institutions that sustain a flourishing practice

'No practices can survive for any length of time unsustained by institutions', states MacIntyre with confidence.[1] This is obviously true for health care, which has always been supported by institutions, from the Aesculapium of ancient Kos through medieval monasteries with their infirmaries and herb gardens, to the charitable hospitals of the eighteenth and nineteenth centuries. As practices develop, typically their institutional forms change. As the practice of health care has grown more complex, particularly in the last century, its institutions have also grown more complex. In the mid-nineteenth century the rather individualistic profession of medicine was complemented by nursing, a more collaborative profession working in structured teams within the practice, which made possible the transformation of hospitals from lodging houses for the sick to places of care and healing.

The twentieth century has seen further growth of teams, both within and outside hospitals. They now involve other health professions and managers as well as doctors and nurses, each of whom bring their particular virtues and vices, make their peculiar contribution to the practice's purpose, gain their own internal goods and cultivate their peculiar virtues – though there is a strong family resemblance between the virtues of all professionals involved in health care. Alongside this development in the practice, hospitals have grown into multi-departmental organisations, as complex and hard to organise as any large factory or business. Over the same period general practice has grown from being usually a single doctor, working out of a couple of rooms of his house with basic reception duties and practice administration being just another part of his wife's job of running their home, into multi-doctor, multiprofessional teams with their own premises and a turnover of several million pounds a year, in many respects much more like hospitals than previous institutions supporting primary health care.

The institutions that support health care include not only hospitals, health centres, GP practices and other organisations that house it. Many other institutions also have a largely virtual existence. As health care has grown more complex, bodies have been created to control entry and continuing membership of the professions of medicine, pharmacy, nursing and other health professions; no longer can anyone with the aptitude and inclination take up health care.

Institutions such as the General Medical Council (GMC) and the Nursing and Midwifery Council, whose purpose is to sustain the practice in this respect, have physical bases, but the important part of their support for health care is the policies, regulations and procedures they formulate and implement. Similarly, although we refer to buildings in Euston Road, Regent's Park and Lincoln's Inn Fields as 'royal colleges', the essence of these institutions is their membership and the links the colleges create between them, their corporate activities and the systems that control entry to and continuing membership of these organisations. Their headquarters buildings exist only to house the administrative underpinning of these activities.

The educational structures through which the practice of health care is handed on to new and established professionals are also an important part of the institutional support for health care. They include universities, deaneries, royal colleges and other bodies involved in planning and implementing undergraduate, postgraduate and continuing education for the health professions. Again, whilst some of these (particularly universities) have a very obvious physical presence, less tangible structures such as curricula, teaching programmes and assessment procedures are the more important institutional support that they provide.

The huge cost of modern health care makes state or insurance funding essential. The delivery and control of this funding also involves institutions – the NHS Executive, the Department of Health, health authorities, commissioning groups and health insurance companies, and advisory bodies such as the National Institute for Health and Care Excellence (NICE).

We saw in Chapter 1 examples of how these institutions are structured in terms of different fragments of the moral shipwreck. Regulatory frameworks are conceived mostly in terms of duties and implemented using the tools of managerialism. NICE and other bodies concerned with resource allocation use consequentialist tools like the quality-adjusted life year (QALY). Hospitals, community health organisations and general practices are mainly seen as businesses, driven by the external goods of profit, prestige and ambition. They are factories that produce health care, largely structured by the values of consumerism and managerialism, often seen as amoral systems of fact rather than sets of values.

The example of Mid Staffordshire Hospital

It is impossible to discuss institutions in health care without mentioning the Francis Report,[2] because this is a detailed examination of an institution that spectacularly failed to support a flourishing practice of health care. The report is very clear that, although there were probably individuals who behaved badly, this was primarily an institutional failure. For example, writing in relation to continence and bowel care:

> It is difficult to believe that lapses on the scale that was evidenced could have occurred if there had been an adequately implemented system of nursing and ward management.[3]

And with regard to ensuring patients could eat and drink:

The deficiencies observed in the evidence were not confined to one ward or period. ... There was evidence of unacceptable standards of care as a result of systemic failings. What has been shown is more than can be explained by the personal failings of a few members of staff.[4]

Although some of the problems could be explained in terms of numbers, qualifications, skills and training of staff, the report is clear that there was also a problem of institutional culture. It is worth quoting the paragraph that summarises this in full:

The culture of the Trust was not conducive to providing good care for patients or providing a supportive working environment for staff. A number of factors contributed to this:

- *attitudes of patients and staff – patients' attitudes were characterised by a reluctance to insist on receiving basic care or medication for fear of upsetting staff. Although some members of staff were singled out for praise by patients, concerns were expressed about the lack of compassion and uncaring attitude exhibited by others towards vulnerable patients and the marked indifference they showed to visitors.*

- *bullying – an atmosphere of fear of adverse repercussions in relation to a variety of events was described by a number of staff witnesses. Staff described a forceful style of management (perceived by some as bullying) which was employed on occasion.*

- *target-driven priorities – a high priority was placed on the achievement of targets, and in particular the A&E waiting time target. The pressure to meet this generated a fear, whether justified or not, that failure to meet targets could lead to the sack.*

- *disengagement from management – the consultant body largely dissociated itself from management and often adopted a fatalistic approach to management issues and plans. There was also a lack of trust in management leading to a reluctance to raise concerns.*

- *low staff morale – the constant strain of financial difficulties, staff cuts and difficulties in delivering an acceptable standard of care took its toll on morale and was reflected by absence and sickness rates in particular areas.*

- *isolation – there is a sense that the Trust and its staff carried on much of its work in isolation from the wider NHS community. It was not as open to outside influences and changes in practice as would have been the case in other places and lacked strong associations with neighbouring organisations.*

- *lack of openness – before obtaining Foundation Trust status, the Board conducted a significant amount of business in private when it was questionable whether privacy was really required. One particular incident concerning an attempt to persuade a consultant to alter an adverse report to the coroner has caused serious concern and calls into question how candid the Trust was prepared to be about things that went wrong.*

- *acceptance of poor standards of conduct – evidence suggests that there was an unwillingness to use governance and disciplinary procedures to tackle poor performance. The Inquiry has heard of particular incidents of apparent misconduct which were not dealt with appropriately, promptly or fairly.*

- *reliance on external assessments – The evidence indicates that the Trust was more willing to rely on favourable external assessments of its performance rather than on internal assessment. On the other hand when unfavourable external information was received, such as concerning mortality statistics, there was an undue acceptance of procedural explanations.*

- *denial – In spite of the criticisms the Trust has received recently, there is an unfortunate tendency for some staff and management to discount these by relying on their view that there is much good practice and that the reports are unfair.*[5]

Virtue and vice in institutions

The Francis Report does not use the terms virtue and vice; being mostly written by lawyers and managers not used to thinking in terms of virtue ethics, it would have been surprising if it had done so (although it is perhaps desirable that they should begin to think in such terms). Much of their analysis, however, can be understood in terms of vices or absence of virtue. Bullying of other staff, lack of compassion for patients and relatives, and 'lack of openness' (a managerio-legal euphemism for dishonesty) are obviously vices, but other factors they identify that are less obviously vices are due to absence of essential virtues. Denial of problems is partly the result of lack of *phronesis* and honesty, but also reflects lack of courage, as does the unwillingness to address poor performance or to undertake audit.

Note too that it was not only professionals who needed but lacked courage – the reluctance of patients to insist on receiving basic care or medication for fear of upsetting staff is a courage issue too. This demonstrates that virtue is not just a personal quality – virtue and vice are infectious. In an institution where professionals had allowed a vicious culture of fear, lack of compassion and lack of empathy to develop, only exceptionally courageous patients would be able to point out to staff that they haven't had their medication or their water-jug needed filling. Conversely, if things like this are overlooked (as will happen occasionally even in the best of organisations) if an institution is flourishing in an atmosphere of trust, hope and love, patients will feel able to point this out. The reminder will be acted upon with an automatic apology and the problem will be dealt with.

In the last chapter it was noted that the virtues are commonly held to be indivisible, and they mutually reinforce each other in a 'virtuous circle'. This is probably true for communities as well as individuals – particularly communities engaged in a shared practice like health care. If a community has one virtue then it is more likely to have others; conversely one vice leads to another – not just a slippery slope but a vicious circle. For example, falsifying target records is not only a failure in honesty that makes future dishonesty easier, but also the detachment and denial that people often use to cope with dishonesty erodes caring and empathy. Virtues are to a considerable extent indivisible between individuals too. It is much harder to be virtuous when surrounded by those who are not – there was probably something in those old-fashioned warnings about 'keeping bad company'. The Francis Report gives examples[6] of people feeling pressurised to do wrong against their better judgement. Conversely, it is much easier to develop the habits of acting rightly in a culture where these are the norm.

Institutions that cultivate virtue

The idea that healthcare institutions exist to support the cultivation of the virtues and that without the virtues they cannot succeed in sustaining health care as a flourishing practice may seem strange, but events in Mid Staffordshire illustrate how this is so. This should not surprise us:

The integrity of a practice causally requires the exercise of the virtues by at least some of the individuals who embody it in their activities; conversely the corruption of institutions is always in part at least the effect of the vices.[7]

MacIntyre argues that the chief end of institutional frameworks must be to support the production of the internal goods of the practice; in the case of healthcare institutions this is the health and care of individual patients, which Francis states is the only purpose of a hospital. An axiom of MacIntyre's theory is that to produce these goods we need virtuous, flourishing people. Institutions therefore must help practitioners cultivate the virtues and flourish, so that through their flourishing practice they enable patients to flourish.

Many healthcare institutions already appear to do this. As I argued in Chapter 2, health care is not a practice that is dead, only somewhat damaged and distorted by the moral fragmentation of our society. Despite the criticisms that can be made of the existing institutions sustaining health care, they still do much to support the cultivation of the virtues and enable patients and professionals to flourish, albeit sometimes inadvertently and despite rather than because of their institutional frameworks and policies. Even in an institution as damaged as the Mid Staffordshire Foundation Trust some patients who gave evidence to the Francis Inquiry praised the care that they had received; and many who were critical remained committed to their local hospital and wanted it to succeed.

It seems therefore that the tradition does remain partially intact, and thus a move towards a focus on the virtues and flourishing requires reform and renewal, not revolution. By MacIntyre's perspective any reform of healthcare institutions should be measured against whether or not they contribute to human flourishing and the cultivation of the virtues, primarily for patients but also for professionals, because the production of the internal goods of health for patients requires a community of flourishing professionals.

Unfortunately MacIntyre says very little about what institutions that promote flourishing would look like; certainly he does not offer criteria against which we can evaluate existing institutions. Similarly, although following the Francis Report there is the beginning of a literature on flourishing institutions, so far this is scanty. More than other sections of this work, therefore, the ideas put forward below have to be based largely on my personal experience, which may be atypical; and my interpretation of what I have seen, which may be flawed. The thoughts below should therefore be seen as tentative suggestions by one individual about what may be wrong with our current institutions and ideas on how they might be improved, rather than being the result of wide consultation and a general consensus, as a policy of institutional reform should be.

Institutions that don't help professionals flourish

Healthcare organisations do not always seem to promote flourishing professionals. The focus of the Francis Inquiry[8] was on the concerns of patients and their families, and the experience of professionals played a subsidiary role in the report. Nevertheless, it is clear from Section C, which reports the experiences and perceptions of staff, that for many of them the Mid Staffordshire Foundation Trust did not promote flourishing. Bullying has already been mentioned, but the culture also impaired professionalism; they were working in a 'system that may well have ground down a conscientious practitioner into a seriously pressurised man'.[9] One nurse describes how she was encouraged by colleagues to lie about waiting times in A&E,[10] and their negative response when she refused to do this. The report of her statement makes clear that this impaired her flourishing – even though she responded to the challenge with the courage to say no.

It seems likely that these problems are not confined to Staffordshire. As a GP I have seen a steady trickle of practitioners in health care (and also in education and social work) who feel unsupported, even abused by those who manage their institution. Expectations of workload are sometimes unrealistic, and institutions that exist to promote flourishing in their patients, students or clients fail to take it seriously amongst their professionals. Legal and managerial structures used to investigate complaints and mistakes can be drawn out and adversarial, despite the consensus that dealing with problems effectively requires a 'no blame culture'.[11] Nor is bullying or hostility from colleagues unknown. Such situations can lead to illness, stress related to overwork or burnout. Because typically practitioners in health care, education and social work have a well-developed sense of responsibility, they often feel guilty if they need to take time off, which makes things worse.

Of course my experience is distorted; just as we only have inquiries into hospitals with problems, so a GP only sees the cases where things go wrong. No doubt thousands of instances of illness and critical events in healthcare institutions are handled supportively in ways that promote the growth of all those involved. But we need to examine our institutions to ensure that this is always the case.

Perverse institutions – the European Working Time Directive

The situations discussed above are the outcome of vice or lack of virtue – usually a matter of ignorance or weakness, but occasionally of deliberately vicious actions. But institutional arrangements designed with the best of intentions can also sometimes interfere with the virtuous exercise of professionalism in pursuit of the internal goods of the practice – the perverse incentive.

Pemberton[12] gives an example of this in the story of 'Ruby' – a junior doctor who at the end of her shift is asked to see a patient whose blood pressure is dangerously low. 'How could I say no?' asks Ruby? Quite. But according to the European Working Time Directive (EWTD) she should have said no. Hospitals are required to ensure that their rotas comply with the directive, and they are penalised financially if they fail to meet its requirements. Managers therefore are obliged to make doctors go home when it is time to do so even if the needs of patients require that they stay: 'The New Deal … requires absolute, total compliance, and if one doctor works just half an hour over the stipulated time the entire rota is deemed to have "breached" with severe financial penalties.' So if they stay when emergencies like that facing Ruby arise, junior doctors 'risk the wrath of the management and uncertainty about whether they are still covered by hospital indemnity'. Conversely, 'if they keep walking they breach the duty of care they have to patients'. Moral fragmentation in action.

Pemberton points out other negative effects of the EWTD. There is concern that some doctors are not getting sufficient experience to be able to face the challenges they meet. Rotas that allow for adequate medical cover within the requirements of the directive cut across continuity of care for patients and the continuity of professional relationships and corporate sense of responsibility, which he suggests were associated with the traditional medical 'firm'. He may be idealising the past; the stories of lack of continuity and poor relationships between senior and junior doctors my registrars tell me are not that different from my own experiences more than a quarter of a century ago. But even if things are not worse, they could be better.

The EWTD has the laudable aim of preventing workers being exploited by being forced to work excessive hours. This is not only good for them, their health and their family life but also for society as a whole. Allowing workers to do long hours can be cheaper and easier than employing extra staff, reducing the number of jobs for the unemployed. The excessive working hours once common for junior doctors can lead to poor performance and mistakes as a result of fatigue – the importance of temperance in workload was discussed in Chapter 6. No doubt we need something like the EWTD, but the way in which the directive has been implemented, involving a combination of legalism and managerialism, gives little weight to professionalism, individual autonomy and the importance of flourishing and the virtues.

Similar deformation of practice can result from other regulations in hospitals whose purposes might seem admirable, such as the four-hour target for treatment in A&E, or the 18-week target for out-patient treatment. Commitment to targets rather than patient wellbeing, the substitution of means for ends, process for outcome, was specifically identified as part of the problem in the Francis Report.

Perverse institutions in general practice

General practice is protected to some degree by its dispersed nature and its tradition of informality and self-regulation from these forces, and so has perhaps been less affected by this type of initiative than hospital practice. I have not heard of registrars being forced to eject patients from the consulting room and pack up because their shift has ended, though it was suggested in the 2005 General Election that patients were unable to make appointments to see their GP in advance because this would breach access targets.[13]

An area however where there has been concern that institutional arrangements may inadvertently damage the practice of GPs is the Quality and Outcomes Framework (QOF).[14] This was introduced in 2004 as part of a contract revision that replaced a byzantine system of payments, allowances and target payments that had evolved over more than 50 years of NHS general practice. On the whole replacing a complicated, illogical and bureaucratic system with something simpler which used information that practices would be collecting as part of good routine care seemed sensible[15] and much good has resulted. The clinical aspects of the QOF encourage clinicians to do what they ought to be doing in any case, and encourage the development of systems that help this happen – recall systems, computer reminders and so forth. Against this, some data collection targets seem to increase administration without obvious health benefits, though of course recording that problems exist is an essential preliminary to addressing them. Some people are however concerned that the QOF agenda gets in the way of the patient's agenda[16] and is sometimes intrusive in the consultation.[17] Disease-mongering and incentives to treat people near the end of their lives with little benefit were discussed in Chapters 3 and 4.

Like so many institutions supporting health care, the QOF is based on conflicting moral fragments. The clinical aspects are largely consequentialist, seeking overall health gain for the practice population, whilst the organisational and patient experience domains are based on a mixture of consumerist values and a business/market drive to contain costs, the whole being wrapped up in a managerialist package of fairly rigid targets. Practitioners have to try to implement this within a deontological framework provided by the GMC and the legal cautions of their defence society.

Education for flourishing

The moral fragments that influence health care, particularly the business model and consumerism, also affect educational institutions. The most extreme examples of treating students as customers who are always right, such as the university lecturer denied tenure because students didn't like his use of Socratic questioning and group work, even though these are generally seen as good educational practice,[18] seem to come from the USA. But the UK is not immune to this trend. In a discussion of student satisfaction questionnaires[19] Mary Beard argued that whilst teachers should of course know what students feel about their courses, and teaching which is boring is not usually effective, promoting dissatisfaction and discomfort are important elements in education. Many of her ex-students have told her that they learnt most from parts of the course they hated at the time. The aim of a university education is to help people grow, which sometimes means destabilising them, which is not always comfortable. Nor does she find the conventional feedback form with its boxes to tick (a managerialist tool) necessarily the best way to get information that helps her improve her teaching. She found asking students to write a paragraph on a blank sheet of paper was more useful, but data like these can't be used to create league tables, and so they fall outside the tools of managerialism.

If universities are seen as businesses and students as customers, this will have a long-term impact on the practice of health care, because education for healthcare professionals is part of higher education.

New knowledge and ancient wisdom

To enter into a practice is to enter into a relationship not only with its contemporary practitioners, but also with those who have preceded us in the practice, particularly those whose achievements extended the reach of the practice to its present point.[20]

A feature of our society is a fascination with the novel and the new. In politics this results in a relentless emphasis on 'modernisation'. In health care it appears in the emphasis on using the most up-to-date evidence and the latest drugs. Continuing education is often discussed in terms of 'keeping up to date', and older knowledge tends to be overlooked, the assumption being that anything more than a few years old is not worth reading. The internet has inadvertently exacerbated this tendency. When one went to the library to search for knowledge, evidence from several decades' past was likely to be on the shelves, or at least in the stacks. When the internet became our main source of information, material from before the mid-1990s became less easily available and therefore tended to be ignored, although archiving projects are now overcoming this problem to some extent.

New knowledge and new developments are of course important, but equally we should not overlook the wisdom of our forebears and the achievements of those who have preceded us in the practice. If health care is a practice with a history, our education must include a historical dimension. Clinicians must learn from Hippocrates, know about Galen and his humours (if only to understand patients' health beliefs, which are often still rooted in this theory[21]) and the achievements of Harvey, Parkinson and Osler. It is important that the wisdom of those who have extended the reach of the tradition of general practice in the past – people such as Michael and Enid Balint,[22] Will Pickles of Wensleydale,[23] David Widgery[24] and many others now dead – is not lost.

Virtue is the heart of education

If as MacIntyre suggests we achieve the purpose of the practice, the internal good of health discussed in Chapter 3, and the other internal goods that are the fruits of professionalism through the cultivation of the virtues, then they should be at the centre of education. This turns things upside down. At present education is seen mostly in terms of knowledge and skills, often combined as 'competences'. Personal qualities, attitudes and values come a long way behind, despite being a major contributor to clinical disaster and poor practice (and if you doubt this, again just read the Francis Report). This may be because we lack the language to discuss them or the tools to teach and assess them with the same sophistication as knowledge and skills, and because they are harder (although not impossible) to measure.

This does not mean that knowledge and technical skills (including interpersonal skills) are not important; they are a vital part of *phronesis*, practical wisdom. But the cultivation of the virtues must lie at the heart of professional education.

Institutions of assessment

This does not however mean looking at the world through rose-coloured spectacles, ignoring deficiencies and wrongdoing; indeed, the courage and honesty to face up to problems and deal with them is a vital part of professional virtue. Professionals are sometimes far less than virtuous – most often through ignorance or weakness, but occasionally as a result of deliberately vicious actions; all practices must have minimum standards of virtue amongst their practitioners, and ways of making sure that these are observed. Even comparatively unregulated practices such as parenting have systems (care proceedings, social workers, place of safety orders) that try to ensure that no one practises them at less than a minimal standard. This involves assessment and judgement within organisational frameworks and structures, which protect the bottom line of virtuous practice.

These structures need to help us face up to problems and remedy them before they become too serious. Failure to do this was one of the cultural problems identified in the Francis Report. If they are well designed and properly used, many of them, such as audit, critical incident review and complaints procedures, can contribute to the flourishing of individuals and the practice as well as prevent unacceptable evil. But they are unlikely to work in this way if they start with an assumption of vice and create a hermeneutic of suspicion that demoralises the majority of professionals who, despite their faults, are trying to do their best. Psychological research demonstrates that positive reinforcement is more effective than punishment, and similarly in most cases of poor practice (that is, those that are due to ignorance and weakness rather than deliberate viciousness) carrots rather than sticks are more likely to lead to virtuous practice. Like a riding crop they work best if they stimulate practitioners to move in the right direction rather than inflict significant pain, providing sufficient challenge to develop virtue without overwhelming those to whom they are applied, producing counter-productive denial and hostility. Many existing institutions do work in this way, but unfortunately not all of them.

Walking or talking?

In recent years there has been a significant move from assessment based on personal contact to the collection of paper (or more usually electronic) 'evidence' by those being assessed, which they then submit to the relevant authorities and which may or may not be discussed with the assessor. So, for example, at one time in the deanery in which I worked as a GP trainer (Kent, Surrey and Sussex [KSS]) general practices were approved for training by a visiting team. Whilst background documentation was required, the heart of the assessment was a personal encounter with practice staff and direct examination of clinical records and facilities. This has been replaced by a 'self-assessment questionnaire' that trainers complete, providing written 'evidence' to support their claim to competence. I have observed two features of this practice. First, many colleagues whom my peers and I see as competent and even excellent find collecting such evidence disheartening and depressing. One GP trainer described it as 'the worst experience of my life'. Second, most of the 'evidence' is collected by the person herself, so rather than providing independent validation of the claims for competence or excellence made, in fact it is merely specific self-reported incidents to justify a more general self-reported claim. This is perhaps why it demoralises competent people, both because they feel there is a hollowness in this process, but also because they tend to be self-critical and may find deficiencies in their performance that more objective observers might see as adequate.

The same reliance on self-reported statements is seen in the eportfolios that doctors in training use to record their learning and reflect on their clinical experience, and trainees report similar negative feelings about it.[25] Established doctors produce similar 'evidence' for appraisals. For the award of Fellowship of the Royal College of General Practitioners candidates write statements describing their achievements, and even write their own citation for the ceremony.

Judgements based on a collection of documents, structured in a standard way, seem more objective than ones based on observations by flawed and biased individuals. Although assessment visits of training practices and of hospital training posts, trainer reports on their trainees and recommendations of doctors for FRCGP were usually carried out conscientiously by those involved, and there was often a surprising degree of consensus on the decisions made, the data on which they were based were rather 'soft' and not easily scrutinised by others. If there is an atmosphere of trust and everyone accepts the authority of the assessors this raises no problems, but if they are liable to be challenged in the courts then it is much harder. Portfolios provide data that can be independently reviewed if decisions are disputed, and are the type of evidence lawyers are used to dealing with.[26] This is attractive in an increasingly litigious world where judgements of senior colleagues are no longer accepted without question.

Reflection on practice is essential to the cultivation of the virtues needed to flourish as professionals, but preparing these reports too often becomes a tedious chore rather than a valuable learning experience. Those in love with the jargon of managerialism – lining up ducks, and running things up flagpoles to see who salutes – are fond of asking whether those who 'talk the talk' could 'walk the walk'.[26] These methods seem to judge clinicians largely on how well they 'talk the talk'.

Reflection on experience and self-assessment are of great value as formative exercises, but are they valid as summative assessments? All assessments are biased by the prejudices of the assessor; self-assessment requires you to 'blow your own trumpet', collecting evidence that demonstrates how well you do (even if that includes demonstrating how good you are at identifying your faults, like the interview candidate who gives her greatest weakness as being too conscientious). Someone with a high, perhaps inflated opinion of his own abilities may make a better case than someone more aware of his shortcomings. This encourages the vice of pride and discourages the virtue of humility, perhaps depressing those most aware of what they don't know. A large area of conscious incompetence is a mark of excellence – the wiser and more knowledgeable you are, the more you are aware of what you might know but don't. Conversely, a large area of unconscious incompetence is characteristic of the less able.

Because the candidate collects the evidence, these methods takes less assessor time than more direct assessments, and so may seem to be less costly. Whether however this is true if everyone's time were valued equally is not clear. Many doctors say that preparing for their appraisal takes longer each year, and some trainers completing the KSS Deanery self-assessment questionnaire have complained that the time it takes impinges on other clinical and educational work or eats into their private life. Perhaps direct observation of practice might consume no more professional time overall.

Whatever the time implications, this trend makes assessment increasingly impersonal and practitioners more isolated. Instead of discussing patients and performance with colleagues, clinicians sit in front of computers writing reflective accounts or recording what they do. At best doctors discuss some of this proxy evidence with an assessor – sometimes it is merely sent off by email to be reviewed *in absentia.*

Finally there is the problem of validity – the relationship between the talk and the walk. Written examinations were often criticised for being only loosely related to the ability to apply learning in practice; exercises such as three-hour essay papers and the modified essay question formally used in medical qualifying exams, the MRCGP and other postgraduate examinations have increasingly been replaced by assessments more like real-life practice. How closely is the ability to write a reflection or to keep track of your incidental learning related to performance in practice? Are there doctors who can 'talk the talk' but not 'walk the walk' – and vice versa?

Assessments should be as reliable and objective as possible, but they also need to be valid, encourage the good, detect those with problems, avoid professional isolation, and promote collegiality and flourishing practice. It is not clear that the currently fashionable bureaucratic paperchases are the best way to achieve these goals, but it is less obvious how to do it better. Research that takes account of the values and virtues essential to a flourishing practice is needed to find better ways to meet these criteria for a virtuous assessment process.

Management, education and virtue in appraisal and revalidation

Like so many of the institutions we have considered, the appraisal process is based on separate and sometimes conflicting moral fragments. The background to appraisal is management. Performance appraisal (or performance review) is essentially:

> an opportunity for individual employees and those concerned with their performance, typically line managers, to engage in a dialogue about each individual's performance and development, as well as the support required from the manager. While performance appraisal is an important part of performance management, in itself it is not performance management: rather, it is one of the range of tools that can be used to manage performance.[27]

Appraisal is always more difficult in jobs that involve the provision of a general and reactive service, rather than one with clear targets and defined goals. Appraising receptionists is harder than appraising sales-staff, because it is harder to define and measure success. Much clinical practice is reactive so appraising clinicians is always therefore going to be difficult, and this particularly applies to specialties such as general practice where defined targets and goals cover much less of the work than in narrower specialties. This would be true even in the hierarchical organisations that performance management implies. But there is no line management for GP principals, and even for salaried GPs line management is generally pretty loose. Therefore appraisal of GPs is not normally carried out by line managers as part of performance management. Those aspects of GP performance that can in any real sense be said to be performance managed, such as the QOF, are managed outside the appraisal system at practice level. This makes sense, because even from within a practice it is difficult to establish the contribution of individual practitioners to success or failure in meeting QOF targets. So fitting GPs into this management model is always going to be difficult.

But the Department of Health does not see appraisal as a tool of performance management: 'the primary aim of NHS appraisal is to identify personal and professional development needs'.[28] This definition is conceived not in performance management but in educational terms. Appraisal is usually done by someone unrelated to the GP's workplace and with only a general knowledge of the GP's work and working environment. Many of those involved in NHS appraisal come from an educational background and think of the process largely in terms of educational needs assessment. With its focus on personal growth and development in knowledge, skills and attitudes, the educational model is very close to a virtue ethic, and appraisal viewed in this way would fit very well within a MacIntyrean practice (though rather than misuse a management term, pedants like myself would be happier if it were called something that better fits with this model, such as a periodic review of practice and professional development).

There is however an element of performance management in the process, not in terms of agreed goals and targets relevant to the organisation for the forthcoming year, as the only goals that are set are educational, but in identifying those whose personal performance gives cause for concern – the bottom line of performance appraisal properly so-called. Although the Department of Health defines appraisal as a process of formative assessment, it also links it closely to clinical governance.[29] Well done, performance management can help the good to excel, the less good to improve and in a small minority identify the need for remedial or punitive action. Since however the last is the only performance management goal that the GP appraisal process can really achieve, it risks becomes legalistic and imbued with a hermeneutic of suspicion.

Appraisal, largely based on the type of documentation discussed above collected by the appraisee, has been chosen as the basis for revalidation for GPs. This decision has inevitably accentuated the summative aspect of the process. The requirement to provide information in a standard form is another very concrete result of this; a formative educational review does not need such standardisation, but can and should be tailored to the individual. So too is the demoralisation that some practitioners feel when approaching (and sometimes after completing) their appraisal, because if its main purpose is to prove that the doctor's practice is above the minimum standard the emphasis has to be on what is omitted and what is not done well, no matter how much the rhetoric speaks of celebrating good practice. How effective this will be at rooting out poor practice remains to be seen;[30] it is however hard to see how it will help the majority of good and indifferent GPs to greater flourishing to the benefit of their patients.

What types of institutions best sustain flourishing practices?

Analysing how institutions do not promote flourishing practice is comparatively easy. Finding ways in which the good intentions of the institutions critiqued above can be achieved in ways that are more flexible and take account of professionalism, flourishing and the internal goods of practice is more difficult.

MacIntyre points out, 'Without the virtues there could be a recognition only of what I have called the external goods' and 'In any society which recognised only external goods competitiveness would be the dominant and even exclusive feature.'[31] Some of the deficiencies noted, and those which the Francis Report identified, such as an excessive reliance on external assessments and target-driven priorities reflect a commitment to external rather than internal goods. We saw in Chapter 5 how the rewards of professionalism are often seen largely in terms of external goods, and throughout this book how competitiveness and adversarial relationships threaten to dominate health care. If the main purpose of institutions is to support practices in which virtues are cultivated and internal goods produced, it follows that emphasis on external goods and competitiveness are deficiencies of our institutional structures. If health care is to become a flourishing MacIntyrean practice then institutions need to focus on internal goods and encourage collaboration and internal drivers for excellence.

Because practices are collaborative, relationships between practitioners are central and therefore institutional structures need to promote these. On the whole relationships are easier to cultivate and maintain in smaller institutions – as Schumacher put it, 'Small is beautiful'.[32] But this is not the only factor that determines whether institutions support relationships. General practices with three or four partners who rarely talk to each other demonstrate that small can be ugly too! Conversely, large institutions do not have to be impersonal; they can be organised so that people only have to deal with a manageable number of relationships, and so that these are cultivated and cherished. Since many aspects of modern health care are only practicable in large institutions, devising systems that achieve this is essential.

Continuity is important: not only continuity of care between clinician and patient but continuity of relationships between clinicians and between clinicians and managers. Relationships take time to develop, but when they are established they make communication easier and more effective. Financial pressures and an emphasis on cost-effective 'skill mix' also however often make this difficult – sometimes with disastrous results, as was seen in the reorganisation of ward teams into larger 'clinical floors' discussed in the Francis Report.[33] The continuous reform of the NHS in recent decades has not helped continuity of relationships, and some healthcare institutions seem to prefer administrative convenience to continuity of relationships. Several times in my experience health visitors and district nurses who knew and understood their patients, and with whom I and my colleagues had built useful working relationships, have been moved by the institutions that employed them against their will, with little regard to the importance of sustaining relationships and continuity of care.

Some current trends support the development of relationships. GP federations and commissioning groups link clinicians together who previously had little contact. Patient participation groups can promote relationships too, but this needs to be a genuine partnership, not tokenism or consumerism; 'patient engagement' can become another box to tick, most easily solved by involving 'professional patients' who make a hobby or almost a career of this role. They bear the same relationship to the average patient as the theatre critic does to the average theatregoer.

Other recent trends are perhaps less helpful to building relationships. The move from solitary GPs taking calls at home to GP co-ops not only gave patients an awake doctor and doctors an awake life, but it also tended to promote community amongst general practitioners who came out of their silos and worked as a team. The further recent shifts to larger and less personal institutions to provide out-of-hours care risk reversing this trend, although since human relationships flourish and contribute to flourishing even in the worst circumstances some of it still happens.

It is important not to confuse whether an institution is commercial or non-profit making with whether it supports a flourishing practice or not. Organisations with a profit motive can support flourishing so long as internal goods are seen as central and external goods though important as secondary. Conversely non-profit-making organisations with excessive faith in managerialism and legalism can undermine flourishing, because they look for 'systems so perfect that no-one will need to be good'[34] and therefore do not focus on the cultivation of virtues and relationships.

Notes

1. MacIntyre A. *After Virtue: a study in moral theory* (2nd edn). London: Duckworth, 1985, Chapter 14.

2. Francis R. *Independent Inquiry into Care Provided by Mid Staffordshire NHS Foundation Trust: January 2005–March 2009.* Volume 1. London: The Stationery Office, 2013, http://webarchive.nationalarchives.gov.uk/20130107105354/http://www.dh.gov.uk/prod_consum_dh/groups/dh_digitalassets/@dh/@en/@ps/documents/digitalasset/dh_113447.pdf [accessed 16 January 2014].

3. Francis. *Independent Inquiry*, Executive Summary, para. 22

4. Francis. *Independent Inquiry*, Executive Summary, para. 30.

5. Francis. *Independent Inquiry*, para. 40.

6. Francis. *Independent Inquiry*, e.g. para. 29–32.

7. MacIntyre. *After Virtue*, Chapter 14, p. 195.

8. Francis. *Independent Inquiry*, Introduction.

9. Francis. *Independent Inquiry* (*op. cit.*).

10. Francis. *Independent Inquiry* (*op. cit.*).

11. Department of Health. *A Promise to Learn, a Commitment to Act. Improving the Safety of Patients in England.* London: DH, 2013, www.gov.uk/government/publications/berwick-review-into-patient-safety [accessed 5 March 2014].

12. Pemberton M. What is the EU doing to our doctors? *Daily Telegraph*, 9 September 2010, www.telegraph.co.uk/health/7991012/What-is-the-EU-doing-to-our-doctors.html [accessed 16 January 2014].

13. Blair promises action on GP row. *BBC News*, 29 April 2009, http://news.bbc.co.uk/1/hi/uk_politics/vote_2005/frontpage/4495865.stm [accessed 16 January 2014].

14. British Medical Association. *Quality and Outcomes Framework for 2012/13: guidance for PCOs and practices.* London: General Practitioners Committee, www.gpcwm.org.uk/wp-content/uploads/file/QOF/QOF_Guidance_2012_2013_guidance_for_pcos_and_practices_june2012.pdf [accessed 16 January 2014].

15. Toon PD. Burn the red book. 1995. Unpublished paper circulated within the Department of Health and the BMA's General Medical Services Council. Copy available from author on request.

16. Wilmington Health Care Limited. QOF – are GPs stuck on the hamster wheel? Editorial. 20 November 2012. www.onmedica.com/ViewsArticle.aspx?id=c8c9a93d-a667-4d33-a90f-8faca9f408c3 [accessed 16 January 2014].

17. Mitchell C, Dwyer R, Hagan T, *et al.* Impact of the QOF and the NICE guideline in the diagnosis and management of depression: a qualitative study. *British Journal of General Practice* 2011; **61(586)**: e279–e289. ePub 26 April 2011. www.ncbi.nlm.nih.gov/pubmed/21619752 [accessed 16 January 2014].

18. Basu K. Socratic backfire? *Inside Higher Education*, 31 October 2011, www.insidehighered.com/news/2011/10/31/after-student-complaints-utah-professor-denied-job [accessed 16 January 2014].

19. Beard M. *A Point of View: marks out of ten please.* Radio talk, 30 November 2012, www.bbc.co.uk/podcasts/series/pov/all [accessed 16 January 2014].

20. MacIntyre. *After Virtue*, Chapter 14, p. 195.

21. Fuller J, Toon PD. *Medical Practice in a Multicultural Society.* London: Heinemann Professional, 1987.

22. Balint M. *The Doctor, His Patient and the Illness* (2nd edn). London: Livingstone, 1964 [1957].

23. Pemberton J. *Will Pickles of Wensleydale: the life of a country doctor.* London: Geoffrey Bles, 1970.

24. Hutt P. *Confronting an Ill Society: David Widgery, general practice, idealism and the chase for change.* Oxford: Radcliffe, 2004.

25. Stillman K. A service evaluation of the nMRCGP e-portfolio learning log as an educational tool for developing reflexive practice in GP trainees. Thesis submitted in partial fulfilment of the MA requirements, South Bank University, 2012.

26. Martin G. Walk the walk. *The Phrase Finder,* www.phrases.org.uk/meanings/walk-the-walk.html [accessed 16 January 2014].

27. CIPD. Performance appraisal: resource summary. 2013. www.cipd.co.uk/subjects/perfmangmt/appfdbck/perfapp.htm?IsSrchRes=1 [accessed 16 January 2014].

28. Department of Health. Appraisals. 2010. http://webarchive.nationalarchives.gov.uk/+/www.dh.gov.uk/en/Managingyourorganisation/Workforce/EducationTrainingandDevelopment/Appraisals/DH_446 [accessed 20 October 2013].

29. KPMG Working Group on Medical Revalidation and Education. *Review of the Readiness of Appraisal and Clinical Governance to Support the Relicensure of Doctors.* Commissioned by the Department of Health and the General Medical Council. London: DH, 2008.

30. Toon P, Swinglehurst D, Shale S, *et al.* Exploring the relationship between professionalism and revalidation. The Christmas Colloquium 2012, Linkedin Primary Care Ethics Forum. www.linkedin.com/groupItem?view=&gid=4315768&type=member&item=196626559&qid=e4d3a210-8a46-4c3b-a98a-6e8eab734dc0&goback=%2Eanp_4315768_1382341463792_1%2Egmr_4315768%2Egna_4315768 [accessed 16 January 2014].

31. MacIntyre. *After Virtue*, Chapter 14.

32. Schumacher EF. *Small Is Beautiful: economics as if people mattered.* New York: Harper & Row, 1973.

33. Francis. *Independent Inquiry (op. cit.)*

34. Eliot TS. Choruses from the Rock [1934]. In: *Complete Poems and Plays.* London: Faber & Faber, 1972.

Chapter 8

Towards a flourishing practice

A partial solution

Alasdair MacIntyre modestly claimed that *After Virtue* was a partial solution[1] to the moral fragmentation he believed underlied many of our society's problems. If this is true then this attempt to apply his ideas to health care is not even a partial solution; it is at best a signpost to a road worth exploring and a few hints on where that road might lead. There is much more to be said on how participation in health care helps patients cultivate the virtues necessary for flourishing, to live a good life and have a good death. Fortunately there is already a large literature that, although not phrased in terms of virtues and flourishing, nevertheless has much to teach us about these issues.

Sadly the same cannot be said about how we use disease concepts to promote the flourishing of the individual, where much of what has been written consists of rhetoric shouted from different fragments of the moral shipwreck. A lot more work on the issues raised in Chapter 4 is important if health care is to become a more flourishing practice.

The debate on professional values and professionalism also seems to have got rather stuck.[2] Perhaps reconceptualising it in terms of virtue and flourishing may help unblock this, since this is also partly the result of incommensurable moral fragments becoming impacted. Here too many contributions to the existing discussion fit well within the framework I have proposed, and provide a good basis for a far more developed and nuanced account of professionalism than I have been able to offer.

There is a temptation to see the solution to the problems we face primarily in terms of institutional reform, and in recent years the mania for addressing problems by reorganisation (a consequence of embracing the 'faith of the managers'[3]) has become almost a joke. Whilst no doubt many institutions supporting health care do need reform to help them better support the practice, this must start from a consideration of virtues and internal goods. MacIntyre is very clear: 'The ability of a practice to retain its integrity will depend on the way in which the virtues can be and are exercised in sustaining the institutional forms which are the social bearers of the practice' and 'The corruption of institutions is always in part at least an effect of the vices'.

So if we want to change our institutions so that they sustain health care as a flourishing practice we need to start not by thinking about reorganisation but about the practice. Only if our practice focuses on the virtues and its internal goods will we be in a position to change our institutions so they better support a flourishing practice. The key criterion against which any healthcare reform should be tested is 'Does it contribute to human flourishing and the cultivation of the virtues for both patients and practitioners, or is it detrimental to these?'

It is often suggested that important factors in health care like virtue and flourishing cannot be measured, but this is false. 'If something exists, it exists in some quantity, and if it exists in some quantity then it can be measured.'[4] Meaningful measurement of complex factors is not easy, but psychology offers us many sophisticated approaches to measurement not currently widely used. Finding ways to measure what is important rather than settling for measuring what is easy is an important step towards a more flourishing practice.

Just as the idea that institutions exist primarily to cultivate the virtues is unfamiliar, it is hard for us to think of the problems our institutions face as due to 'vices'. These days this word tends to be used either of trivial weakness (excessive fondness for cream cakes and chocolate that are 'naughty but nice') or the extreme of deliberate evil (vice-rings). In reality most vice lies between these two extremes. Much of it is not deliberate as much as misguided. Virtue is both the habit of acting rightly but also is according to reason,[5] and *phronesis* lies at the heart of the virtues. Its absence is just as much a vice as the more obvious sins of greed, ambition and selfishness. Perhaps it might be better if we adopted Urmson's suggestion and translated *arete* as 'excellence' rather than 'virtue'.[6]

Tradition and change

Because of MacIntyre's emphasis on a tradition that goes back to Aristotle and Aquinas, and his accusation that many of our problems stem from the Enlightenment that ushered in modernism, there is a risk that an ethical framework based on his work could be backwards looking, a sort of philosophical Arts and Crafts Movement harking nostalgically after simpler, earlier days, perhaps looking for a return to the 'traditional professionalism' characterised in the documents discussed in Chapter 5. This is not what we need. A move towards a practice flourishing in the way MacIntyre would approve of might involve reversing some recent trends, such as excessive emphasis on markets, consumerism, legal and managerial regulation. But equally it would mean encouraging others: patient–clinician partnership, explicit discussion of values, teamwork and the valuing of other professionals as well as doctors. Fashionable concepts like integrated care[7] with its emphasis on different professionals working together with patients to provide a better outcome would seem likely to move health care towards being a flourishing practice. The emphasis on the importance of a holistic view and agreeing plans with patients in GP training,[8] and the narrative medicine movement,[9] are other examples of ways in which we are already moving towards a practice centred on flourishing narratives and virtues.

What to do with the fragments

This exploration started with a consideration of how the fragments of the moral shipwreck affect health care, and if health care is to become a flourishing practice then we must find a way to integrate them into a coherent moral framework which fulfils the functions that they attempt. Some of this is fairly straightforward. Deontological frameworks can be recast in terms of the virtues, as the statement of the 'Virtues of the Doctor' (see Box 8.1 on pp. 124–5) based on the GMC's deontological statement of values demonstrates. A similar process can be undertaken with other parts of the institutional framework currently cast in terms of rights and duties. It takes a while to change a mind-set frozen in terms of Kantian deontology but it can be done.

Dealing with managerialism too is straightforward, at least in theory. It certainly does not mean getting rid of managers – often a popular scapegoat when things go wrong. Sacking managers without changing the way a service is organised just leads to badly managed (and therefore inefficient) health care. Managers are an important part of the practice of health care, and are not necessarily any more afflicted by managerialism than clinicians (or even patients). We can continue to benefit from the tools of management if they are kept in their proper place; a means to safe patient care, the cultivation of virtue and flourishing rather than ends in themselves.

Rosen and Dewar were concerned about the danger that appraisal and revalidation 'could become administrative exercises rather than a regular opportunity to review and reflect upon how far each doctor's clinical practice measures up to the standards of good medical practice',[10] a prophecy that many doctors would feel has already been fulfilled. But this does not mean we should abandon appraisal or revalidation. We need to examine management structures and ensure that managerialist values do not trump others that are more important. This needs to be a collaborative process – we must be careful that this does not develop into a tussle between managers and clinicians for the control of health care. The Francis Report[11] is an excellent starting point for this process.

The analysis above however suggests that consumerism is a snare and a delusion. Seeing health care as a collaborative activity involving patients and professionals in partnership is a far more helpful way to put patients at the centre of our thinking and promote their autonomy than consumerism. Similarly there are ways to stimulate excellence and contain costs without relying primarily on the dogma of the market and on external goods.

Overcoming legalism is difficult, not only because of the grip that legal thinking has over so many areas of our society, including health care, but also because we do need legal frameworks as part of the institutional support for health care, and it may be harder to untangle legalism and the law than management from managerialism. But our laws too need to be conceptualised and implemented so as to promote flourishing. This might however require a change in the thinking of lawyers, which is perhaps hard to envisage.

The need for justice

As the costs of health care continue to rise, a satisfactory account of the virtue of justice is essential. This needs to be robust enough to do the tasks for which we currently use consequentialism. It is fairly easy to move from conceptualising what has to be done for an individual from maximising pleasure to promoting a flourishing narrative, and so to imagine what it means to act justly towards individual patients in this context. But health care consumes enormous resources (8.7% of GDP in the UK in 2008)[12] and consequentialism is the main tool used to make resource allocation policy. Finding a theory of justice that aims at flourishing to replace the blunt instrument of consequentialism is perhaps the greatest challenge for a MacIntyrean approach to health care. Can we develop a set of v-rules[13] that help us to make just policy decisions on how we spend our money?

We also need a just approach to the distribution of external goods to professionals in health care. The focus of a flourishing practice must be on internal goods and the cultivation of the virtues, but if professionals are to focus on producing its internal goods they do need an income sufficient to remove the worry of where the next meal is coming from. Almost everyone has to earn a living, and virtuous practice in other parts of our lives – as parents, carers, spouses and so on – requires that professionals earn the money they need to carry out those roles effectively. For many professionals in health care this currently is the case, but for some it is not, and for others who earn enough for their need unfortunately greed (excessive desire for material external goods) or lust for non-material external goods such as power, prestige and fame can interfere with focusing on the internal goods. The continual emphasis on the importance of external goods in our consumerist, celebrity-obsessed society makes it hard for even those whose natural inclination is towards internal goods to avoid being sucked into these vices.

Where next?

There is clearly much thinking to do to bring the fragments of our moral discourse together. This will need collaboration between philosophers and practitioners (both professionals and patients), for a single group cannot solve the problems alone. As well as taking further some of the issues I have discussed, there is work to be done on issues I have barely mentioned. Developing genuine collaboration between patients and professionals requires more thought, but also much more action. Politicians and other 'stakeholders' have to be persuaded of the virtue of virtue if we are to move towards a coherent, unified practice of health care. When the Head of the Professional Standards Authority calls upon the health professions to find their moral purpose, there are however grounds for optimism that our society is ready for the sort of paradigm shift that embracing a MacIntyrean perspective would involve.[14]

Health care is just one aspect of society, and some of the ideas discussed above have ramifications far beyond our practice. This may make implementing them a challenge, but it is encouraging that many of the problems affecting health care have also been identified in other practices, particularly education, but also in the business community as a result of the banking crisis of 2008 and subsequent events. Perhaps health care can lead the way towards a society more generally oriented to flourishing.

MacIntyre suggested that overcoming the fragmentation of moral discourse that arose at the Enlightenment will require 'a new and no doubt very different St Benedict'.[15] I am not sure he is right. The solution to the problems we currently face will probably not come from some towering innovative figure; to look for such a solution is to buy into the obsession with celebrity and centralised solutions that dominate our society. I think it is more likely to come from thousands of ordinary practitioners putting the cultivation of the virtues at the heart of their practice and making many small changes in how we work and how we organise ourselves that over time will heal our damaged practice. All everyone needs to do is to start doing this.

Box 8.1: Virtues or duties?

The virtues of a doctor registered with the General Medical Council*	The duties of a doctor registered with the General Medical Council
The practice of medicine can be an extremely fulfilling way to spend one's life, but it is not easy. Sincerely undertaken with the support of your colleagues, however, through its study and practice you will be able to develop the personal qualities needed to succeed in your chosen profession. We summarise these qualities in key attributes, which we call the virtues of a doctor – the personal qualities that are both needed for and are the reward of good medical practice.	Registration carries both privileges and responsibilities. We summarise these responsibilities in 14 key principles, which we call the duties of a doctor – the contract between doctor and patient that is at the heart of medicine.
All doctors must have:	Patients must be able to trust doctors with their lives and wellbeing. To justify that trust, we as a profession have a duty to maintain a good standard of practice and care, and to show respect for human life.
• the concentration to focus attention fully on the problems of the patient	In particular as a doctor you must:
• the patience to treat every patient politely and considerately	• make the care of your patient your first concern
• the trustworthiness and discretion needed to handle access to patients in private and intimate situations	• treat every patient politely and considerately
• the patience and understanding to listen to patients' stories and appreciate their viewpoints	• respect patients' dignity and privacy
• the clarity to explain complicated ideas to patients in a simple way.	• listen to patients and respect their views
Medicine offers:	• give patients information in a way they can understand
• the privilege of standing alongside people as they face the most important challenges in their lives	• respect the rights of patients to be fully involved in decisions about their care
• the opportunity to collaborate with people as they make decisions about their health and their life	• keep your professional knowledge and skills up to date
• the chance to be a lifelong learner, always growing and developing as a doctor and as a person.	• recognise the limits of your professional competence
	• be honest and trustworthy
	• respect and protect confidential information
	• make sure that your personal beliefs do not prejudice your patients' care
	• act quickly to protect patients from risk if you have good reason to believe that you or a colleague may not be fit to practise
	• avoid abusing your position as a doctor
	• work with colleagues in the ways that best serve patients' interests.

The virtues of a doctor registered with the General Medical Council*	The duties of a doctor registered with the General Medical Council
To succeed as a doctor you will need: • the humility to acknowledge your own limitations • honesty and trustworthiness • the wisdom to keep confidential information secret • the justice to prevent your personal beliefs prejudicing your patients' care • the courage to act quickly to protect patients from risk if you have good reason to believe that you or a colleague may not be fit to practise • the temperance to avoid abusing your position as a doctor • the spirit of cooperation to work with colleagues to benefit you, your colleagues and your patients. Acquiring the fullness of these virtues is a life's work (*ars longa, vita brevis*), but if you engage earnestly in your medical studies you will have them to a sufficient degree on registration for medical practice to be a safe and fulfilling profession for you and your patients. If you practise sincerely, as time goes by you will, with the support of your colleagues and your patients, grow in the richness of these virtues and become a better doctor for you and for your patients.	In all these matters you must never discriminate unfairly against your patients or colleagues. And you must always be prepared to justify your actions to them.

* This catalogue is an attempt to provide a virtue parallel to the GMC's 'Duties of a doctor' for illustrative purposes. It does not imply that these are the only virtues needed by doctors or that a virtue-based definition of the qualities a doctor needs should necessarily mirror the GMC's duties so closely.

Notes

1. MacIntyre A. *After Virtue: a study in moral theory* (2nd edn). London: Duckworth, 1985, p. 201.

2. Christmas S, Millward L. *New Medical Professionalism.* A scoping report for the Health Foundation. London: Health Foundation, 2011, www.health.org.uk/public/cms/75/76/313/2733/New%20medical%20professionalism.pdf?realName=JOGEKF.pdf accessed [accessed 16 January 2013].

3. Pattison S. *Faith of the Managers: when management becomes religion.* London: Cassell, 1997.

4. A favourite saying of Mal Salkind, a former Professor of General Practice and Primary Care at Queen Mary University of London.

5. Aquinas, St Thomas. *Summa Theologica.* Cambridge: Cambridge University Press, 1990; Latin original and English translation, www.sacred-texts.com/chr/aquinas/summa/sum191.htm [accessed 16 January 2014].

6. Aristotle. *The Ethics of Aristotle: the Nicomachean ethics* (trans. JAK Thomson). Harmondsworth: Penguin, 1955.

7. The King's Fund. Integrated care. 2012. www.kingsfund.org.uk/topics/integrated-care [accessed 16 January 2014].

8. Royal College of General Practitioners. MRCGP Clinical Skills Assessment CSA candidate feedback for exams taken from January 2012. Statement 12. Does not appear to develop rapport or show awareness of patient's agenda, health beliefs and preferences. 2012. www.rcgp.org.uk/gp-training-and-exams/mrcgp-exam-overview/~/media/Files/GP-training-and-exams/MRCGP-Clinical-Skills-Assessment-Jan-2012.ashx [accessed 16 January 2014].

9. Launer J. *Narrative-Based Primary Care: a practical guide.* London: Radcliffe, 2002.

10. Rosen R, Dewar S. *On Being a Doctor: redefining medical professionalism for better patient care.* London: King's Fund, 2004, www.kingsfund.org.uk/publications/being-doctor-medical-professionalism [accessed 16 January 2013].

11. Francis R. *Independent Inquiry into Care Provided by Mid Staffordshire NHS Foundation Trust: January 2005–March 2009. Volume 1.* London: The Stationery Office, 2013, http://webarchive.nationalarchives.gov.uk/20130107105354/http://www.dh.gov.uk/prod_consum_dh/groups/dh_digitalassets/@dh/@en/@ps/documents/digitalasset/dh_113447.pdf [accessed 16 January 2014].

12. World Health Organization. *World Health Statistics Part II: global health indicators.* Geneva: WHO, 2011, www.who.int/gho/publications/world_health_statistics/EN_WHS2011_Part2.pdf [accessed 16 January 2014]. See Table 7 'Health expenditure'.

13. Hursthouse R. *Applying Virtue Ethics: study guide* (Open University course A432). Buckingham: Open University, 2000, Part II § 6.

14. Dominiczak P. Mid Staffs scandal: who buried the damning NHS reports? *Daily Telegraph,* 8 March 2013, www.telegraph.co.uk/health/put-patients-first/9917029/Mid-Staffs-scandal-who-buried-the-damning-NHS-reports.html [accessed 16 January 2014].

15. MacIntyre. *After Virtue,* p. 261.

Glossary

The glossary gives some background information and links for further reading about some of some of the key people, ideas and institutions referred to in the book.

People

Aquinas

Born in 1225 in Italy, Thomas Aquinas is probably the most important thinker of the medieval period in Western Europe. His philosophy, known as Thomism, has been influential ever since and is an important source for MacIntyre's thinking. The best known of his writings is the *Summa Theologiæ* (Summary of Theology), a massive work that deals with topics in both theology and philosophy, disciplines that were closely intertwined at that time.

To read more visit: http://plato.stanford.edu/entries/aquinas.

Aristotle

Aristotle was born in 384 BC in Macedonia. He studied at the Academy in Athens under Plato, with whom he competes for the title of most influential Western philosopher ever. After Plato's death he left Athens and researched biology in Asia Minor and Lesbos until Philip of Macedonia appointed him to be tutor to his son, the future Alexander the Great. Aristotle later established another philosophical school in Athens, the Lyceum, where he taught for 13 years until he left the city in 323 BC to avoid political persecution. He died a year later.

He wrote on a wide variety of subjects including physics, linguistics, biology, political science, rhetoric, logic, metaphysics and ethics. Many of his works later became the basis of academic disciplines the scope of which his work had defined. His views on philosophy (particularly logic) and the physical and biological sciences were central to medieval scholarship. His *Ethics* has received increased interest recently with the revival of virtue ethics, and many modern virtue ethicists would describe themselves as Aristotelians.

To read more visit: http://plato.stanford.edu/entries/aristotle.

Balint

Michael Balint was a Hungarian psychoanalyst who fled to England in 1938 to escape the Nazis. In 1945 he obtained a position at the Tavistock Institute, a centre for the study and practice of psychoanalysis in London. In the 1950s with his wife Enid he began to run case discussion groups for GPs. They developed a method based on psychoanalytic theory that used the feelings generated in the doctor and in the discussion group to help understand the doctor–patient relationship and hence the patient's problems better. This work was described in his book *The Doctor, His Patient and the Illness*, which explored aspects of patient behaviour that cannot be understood within the rationalist framework of the medical model, and the therapeutic role of 'the drug doctor'. His ideas were developed further by others through the Balint Society, and were important in the development of the understanding of the doctor–patient relationship in general practice in the UK. Balint groups are now used throughout the world as a learning method not only by GPs but also by psychiatrists, medical students, social workers and lawyers.

To read more visit: http://balint.co.uk.

Benedict of Nursia

Commonly thought of as the founder of Western monasticism, Benedict was born the son of a Roman nobleman in Nursia around AD 480. In his late teens he abandoned his life as a student for a solitary life of prayer and contemplation. His holiness attracted others to him and he founded monasteries, initially at Subiaco and later at Monte Cassino where he died in AD 543.

His vision of monastic life in a community dedicated to prayer, work and study is laid out in his book known as the *Rule of St Benedict*. Monasteries based on his vision were crucial in maintaining a tradition of scholarship in Western Europe through the tumultuous centuries that followed his death, particularly by copying manuscripts of both Christian and pagan authors from antiquity. His insightful and practical *Rule* still governs the life of many Christian religious communities.

To read more visit: www.osb.org/gen/benedict.html.

Buber

Martin Buber (1878–1965) was an Austrian-born Jewish thinker of the twentieth century. Much of his work was in the area of Jewish culture and Zionism. He is however probably best known now for his short philosophical work *Ich und Du* (I and Thou) in which he distinguishes between relationships in which the other, whether that be another person, a plant, an animal or God, is seen as an object (I-It) from I-Thou relationships of encounter or meeting with another unique being. He argued that these two types of relationship reflect two different modes of being that affect us deeply: 'The I of the basic word I-Thou is different from that of the basic word I-It' and 'through the Thou a person becomes I'.

To read more visit: www.iep.utm.edu/buber.

Eliot

Thomas Sterns Eliot was a poet of the twentieth century. Born in St Louis, the United States, he moved to England in his twenties. His first major work, *The Waste Land* (1922), is widely considered to be one of the most important poems of the twentieth century in English, despite its complex structure and diverse, sometimes obscure allusions. He worked for the publisher Faber & Faber and wrote both plays and poetry. Apart from *The Waste Land*, probably his best-known works today are *Murder in the Cathedral*, a play depicting the last days of the life of Thomas Becket, the Archbishop of Canterbury killed on the instructions of King Henry II, and *Four Quartets*, a cycle of four poems each in five 'movements'. He won the Nobel Prize for Literature in 1948 and died in 1965.

To read more visit: www.nobelprize.org/nobel_prizes/literature/laureates/1948/eliot-facts.html.

Heath

Iona Heath was until recently a GP in North London and has been President of the Royal College of General Practitioners. She is one of the leading European thinkers on the nature of general practice, which she has explored in many lectures and articles, particularly in the *British Medical Journal* and in an important monograph, *The Mystery of General Practice*. She has also been prominent in building links between GPs in different countries.

To read more visit: www.nuffieldtrust.org.uk/sites/files/nuffield/publication/The_Mystery_of_General_Practice.pdf.

Hursthouse

Rosalind Hursthouse is a moral philosopher who taught for many years at the Open University in England and now works at the University of Auckland, New Zealand. She has made important contributions to the practical application of virtue ethics, particularly her idea of 'v-rules' – general principles that guide the action of virtuous people. Unlike Kantian principles these are not universal laws; there are occasions when faced with a moral dilemma that a virtuous person will break them, albeit sometimes with regret or even guilt at so doing. She explains her neo-Aristotelian approach to virtue ethics in her book *On Virtue Ethics*, and explores how it works out in practice in her paper 'Virtue theory and abortion'.

To read more visit http://www.debatechamber.com/wp-content/uploads/2010/07/hursthouse-on-abortion.pdf.

Kant

Immanuel Kant (1724–1804) was a German philosopher of the Enlightenment. He is often considered to be the most important philosopher of the modern era and his ideas are the foundation of much nineteenth- and twentieth-century thinking. His philosophy is based on the principles of rationalism, empiricism and human autonomy; he believed that by reason human beings can achieve knowledge and right action. His best-known works are the *Critique of Pure Reason* and the *Critique of Practical (or applied) Reason*. Central ideas in his ethical philosophy were 'the categorical imperative' – that one should act on that principle which one would wish to be a universal law – and also that one should treat people not as means but as ends. This is sometimes popularly paraphrased as 'do as you would be done by'. These principles led him to a deontological ethical theory.

To read more visit: www.rep.routledge.com/article/DB047.

Kuhn

Thomas Samuel Kuhn (1922–96) was one of the most influential philosophers of science of the twentieth century, largely as a result of his book *The Structure of Scientific Revolutions* (1962). He argued that science does not move forwards in a steady progress; it has periods of stable growth punctuated by revolutions when there is a 'paradigm shift'. Such changes occur when *both* the failure of the existing paradigm to solve important anomalies reaches a critical point *and also* the emergence of a credible alternative paradigm overall offers a better explanation of observed phenomena (although the new paradigm may fail to explain phenomena that were dealt with satisfactorily under the old one – 'Kuhn-loss'). An example of a paradigm shift is the change from Newtonian physics to relativity as a result of the work of Albert Einstein.

To read more visit: http://plato.stanford.edu/entries/thomas-kuhn.

Lewis

Clive Staples Lewis was born in Northern Ireland in 1898. He became a Fellow in English literature at Magdalen College, Oxford, in 1925 and wrote a number of influential works of literary criticism. For many years a vehement atheist, he was converted to Christianity in 1929, an experience he describes in his book *Surprised by Joy*. He later wrote a number of books explaining the philosophy of Christianity in simple terms. He is however probably best known now for his fiction, particularly the *Narnia* series, which has been adapted for film and television. Although written for children the series is clearly grounded in his imaginative understanding of the Christian tradition. He was appointed Professor of Medieval and Renaissance Literature at Cambridge in 1954 where he remained until he died in 1963.

To read more visit: www.cslewis.org.

Lloyd George

David Lloyd George (1863–1945) was a Welsh Liberal politician. Initially a solicitor, he became an MP in 1890 and was Chancellor of the Exchequer from 1908–15. His 'People's Budget' of 1909, his Unemployment Insurance Act and the National Insurance Act (1911) provided for healthcare and invalidity benefits, and laid the foundations of the modern welfare state. The record system introduced under this act became known as 'Lloyd George envelopes' and remained in widespread use in the NHS until they were replaced by computerised medical records.

In 1916 he became Prime Minister of a wartime coalition government that held power until 1922, but produced a split in the Liberal Party. He led the Liberal Party from 1926 to 1931, after which he was an increasingly marginal political figure. He was made Earl Lloyd-George of Dwyfor shortly before his death.

To read more visit: http://global.britannica.com/EBchecked/topic/345191/David-Lloyd-George.

MacIntyre

Born in Glasgow in 1929, Alasdair MacIntyre is widely considered to be one of the most influential philosophers of the twentieth century. He taught philosophy at various UK universities before moving to the United States in 1969 where he has had a distinguished academic career. He is best known for a trilogy of works: *After Virtue* (1981), *Whose Justice? Which Rationality?* (1988) and *Three Rival Versions of Moral Enquiry* (1990). In these three books he seeks in different ways to examine the confused state of contemporary philosophical discourse and to resolve that confusion on the basis of the work of Aristotle and Aquinas.

To read more visit: http://www.iep.utm.edu/p-macint.

Maslow

Abraham Maslow (1908–70) was an American psychologist best known for the theory of 'hierarchy of needs' proposed in his 1943 paper 'A Theory of Human Motivation', published in the *Psychological Review*. He argues that needs can be arranged in a hierarchy, often depicted as a pyramid. Human beings seek first to fulfil the most basic physiological needs for air, food, drink, shelter, warmth, sex and sleep. Safety needs come next, followed by the social needs of affection and love and esteem needs, which include status and respect from self and others. At the top of the hierarchy is 'self actualisation' – self-fulfilment and the realisation of our full potential as human beings.

To read more visit www.simplypsychology.org/maslow.html.

Midgley

Born in 1919 the daughter of an Anglican clergyman, Mary Midgley studied philosophy at Oxford and taught at Newcastle University. She only came to public notice after she published her first book *Beast and Man* at the age of fifty-nine. She has since written widely on ethics, human nature and animal rights. She is a vociferous opponent of reductionism, relativism and scientism.

To read more visit: www.theguardian.com/books/2001/jan/13/philosophy.

Sackett

David Lawrence Sackett (born 1934) is a Canadian medical practitioner and clinical epidemiologist who has taught and researched at McMaster University in Canada and at Oxford University. He is best known as a proponent of evidence-based practice, which he defined as 'the integration of best research evidence with clinical expertise and patient values'. Whilst he argued forcefully for the conscientious, explicit and judicious use of current best evidence in making decisions about the care of individual patients, he is clear that 'evidence based medicine is not "cookbook" medicine' and even excellent external evidence may be inapplicable to or inappropriate for an individual patient.

To read more visit: www.dcscience.net/sackett-BMJ-1996.pdf.

Schumacher

Born in Germany in 1911 Ernst Schumacher studied economics in Germany, England and the United States. He moved to England in 1936 to escape the Nazis. His work for the National Coal Board from 1950 to 1970 is widely considered important in the post-war economic recovery of the UK, but he is now best known for his radical thinking on economics 'as if people mattered', influenced by his study of Buddhism and Catholic social teaching. He founded the Intermediate Technology Development Group and published several books explaining his philosophy including *Small is Beautiful, Good Work* and *A Guide for the Perplexed*. He died of a heart attack in 1977.

To read more visit: www.theguardian.com/politics/2011/mar/27/schumacher-david-cameron-small-beautiful.

Thatcher

Born the daughter of a grocer in Grantham in 1925, Margaret Hilda Thatcher (née Roberts) became an MP in 1959. She ousted Edward Heath as leader of the Conservative Party in 1975, and following their election victory in 1979 became the first woman Prime Minister of Great Britain and Northern Ireland. She won two further elections until a decline in her popularity led to her being forced from office in 1990. Her government was notable for its monetarist economic policies, the privatisation of public utilities and services, and legislation that reduced the power of trade unions, which marked a major shift from the post-war social democratic consensus of previous decades. She died in 2013.

To read more visit: www.margaretthatcher.org.

Ideas and institutions

Aesculapium of ancient Kos

Asklepius (Greek) or Aesculapius (Latin) was the god of healing in the Ancient World and so a healing centre was known as an Aesculapium. The ruins of one such establishment probably dating from the fourth century BC can still be seen on Kos, where the great medical writer Hippocrates is said to have founded the medical school. It seems to have been both a shrine to the god and a place where people went for treatment and for the teaching of medicine – perhaps the ancient equivalent of a modern teaching hospital.

To read more visit: http://kos-greece.net/asklepion.

Choose and Book

This is an internet-based system for booking hospital appointments and other referrals from general practice in the UK. It was introduced in 2005 to replace the traditional system whereby the GP wrote a letter that was posted to the hospital and the patient was then sent an appointment, also by post.

With Choose and Book, when the GP and patient decide that a referral is appropriate they select one or more referral centres from an online list. The patient can then book an appointment him or herself later by phone or online, or the GP and patient can book it together on the spot. A referral letter in electronic form is routed to the appropriate hospital by the software.

Its introduction was marked by the delays and teething troubles often seen with large software projects. Its reception has been mixed and the original intention that it would be used for almost all referrals to hospital has not been realised.

To read more visit: www.chooseandbook.nhs.uk/patients/whatiscab.

Consequentialism

Consequentialist ethical theories take the view that whether an action is right or not depends on its outcome or consequences; the right choice is that action which leads to 'the greatest good of the greatest number'. The implication of this is that 'the end justifies the means'; so for example killing an innocent person by act or omission would be morally right if this prevented the death of a larger number of people. Since not to act is also in one sense an action, consequentialism sees no moral difference between acts and omissions.

The best-known version of consequentialism is utilitarianism, propounded by Jeremy Bentham (1748–1832), which argues that right action maximises pleasure and minimises pain. For Bentham all forms of pleasure were of equal value, but the later utilitarian John Stuart Mill (1806–73) argued that intellectual and moral pleasures are superior to more physical forms of pleasure, and distinguished between happiness and contentment: 'it is better to be a human being dissatisfied than a pig satisfied; better to be Socrates dissatisfied than a fool satisfied'.

There are several other forms of consequentialism that take different views on the nature of the good that is to be maximised. Rule utilitarianism is the view that deciding on the utility of individual acts is impractical, so one should act according to rules that in general tend to lead to the greatest good of the greatest number. National Institute for Health and Care Excellence (NICE) guidance on clinical priorities can be seen as an example of rule utilitarianism, often using an important consequentialist tool, the 'quality-adjusted life year (QALY)', to calculate the consequences of different choices.

To read more visit: http://plato.stanford.edu/entries/consequentialism.

Deontology

Derived from the Greek word *deon*, which means duty, deontological ethical theories are those which hold that certain acts, such as lying, stealing or killing innocent people, are intrinsically wrong. This means, for example, that one should tell the truth even if this leads to harm or even death. A positive duty implies an obligation to act, for example a physician's duty of care. A negative duty implies an obligation to refrain from an action, for example the duty not to steal. Deontological systems have been justified in terms of divine commandment or natural law or as by Immanuel Kant on the basis of principles of human reason.

Deontological theories are also often expressed in terms of rights, which bear a reciprocal relationship to duties – a 'claim' right such as the right to health care implies that someone has a positive duty to fulfil that claim; a 'liberty right' such as freedom of speech implies that everyone has a negative duty not to interfere with the exercise of that right.

To read more visit: http://plato.stanford.edu/entries/ethics-deontological.

Enlightenment

The Enlightenment or the Age of Reason is the period in Western thought and culture in the late seventeenth and eighteenth centuries during which there were dramatic revolutions in science, philosophy, society and politics. Empirical research and philosophy based on reason replaced the medieval world view, while the Enlightenment ideals of freedom and equality for all based on human reason led to the French Revolution and secular republicanism. Enlightenment ideas that continue to influence our society include: body/mind dualism (particularly clearly expounded by René Descartes, and often referred to as Cartesian dualism);

a faith in reason and empiricism rather than tradition, authority or experience as the road to truth; and an optimistic view of the capacity of human reason to achieve progress and growing certainty.

In recent years some of the assumptions of the Enlightenment have been questioned not only by Alisdair MacIntyre but also by a variety of 'postmodernist' thinkers more sceptical about the possibility of absolute knowledge. Others too have questioned the capacity of human reason and take a more pessimistic view of human nature.

To read more visit: http://plato.stanford.edu/entries/enlightenment.

Hermeneutics

In its narrower sense hermeneutics is the theory of how to interpret texts, a term originally mainly used with respect to biblical texts. It is also however now used more widely to encompass the study of all texts, and also by extension other forms of communication, and even philosophical questions as to how and whether we can communicate at all.

Thus for example the 'interpretative function' in which a GP helps patients make sense of their illness in the overall context of their lives can be described as 'the hermeneutic function', helping them to read the story of their 'live narrative'.

The French philosopher Paul Ricœur distinguished between two forms of hermeneutics: a 'hermeneutics of faith', which looks for meaning in a text, and a hermeneutics of suspicion, which looks for disguised meanings and sees reading as decoding. More recently the term has also been used more loosely to describe an approach of extreme scepticism to the veracity and accuracy of any text.

To read more visit: http://plato.stanford.edu/entries/hermeneutics.

New to follow-up ratio

NHS management is concerned that hospitals sometimes follow up out-patients unnecessarily when it would be more cost-effective for them to be discharged. When hospitals are paid according to the work they do then follow-up appointments can add considerably to the cost of treatment (or from the perspective of hospitals add to the income generated!).

For this reason hospital contracts often include targets for the ratio of new patients seen to follow-up appointments, and penalties for exceeding these ratios. First appointments are also often paid at a higher rate than follow-ups. Specialists in chronic diseases that require hospital follow-up such as rheumatology, however, argue that these ratios make no sense in their field as follow-up is a key element in their work, and if they discharge patients they will merely need to be re-referred, which will increase costs as they will then again be 'new patients'.

To read more visit: www.productivity.nhs.uk/PCT_Dashboard and select 'Managing First Follow Up'; or visit www.bmj.com/content/342/bmj.c7373.

NICE

NICE is the body that provides national guidance and advice in the UK to improve health and social care. It was originally set up in 1999 as the National Institute for Clinical Excellence to reduce variation in the availability and quality of NHS treatments and care, as part of the then government's NHS policies outlined in *A First Class Service: quality in the new NHS.*

In 2005 it merged with the Health Development Agency to become the National Institute for Health and Clinical Excellence and began developing public health as well as clinical guidance. In April 2013 it also took on responsibility for developing guidance and quality standards in social care, and its name changed again to the National Institute for Health and Care Excellence, although the acronym NICE is still used.

To read more visit: www.nice.org.uk.

Phronesis

This is the Greek word for the virtue of being able to reason out what is the right action in any particular situation. It is both an intellectual and a moral excellence of character. Traditionally it is translated as prudence in English (via the Latin *prudentia*) and with temperance, courage and justice is one of the four cardinal virtues. It is often now however translated as practical wisdom because prudence has come to imply a cautious attitude, which was not part of the original meaning.

To read more visit: http://grammar.about.com/od/pq/g/Phronesis-term.htm.

QOF

The Quality and Outcomes Framework (QOF) was introduced as part of the reform of the NHS Contract with GPs in the UK in 2004. It provides for payments based on a points system for meeting performance targets on activities that the Department of Health wishes to encourage. These include screening and health promotion activities, the structured care of chronic diseases and practice organisation. The detailed criteria and standards change each year; NICE advises on the clinical content and the whole is negotiated between the NHS and GP representatives.

To read more visit: www.nhshistory.net/gppay.pdf.

Socratic questioning

The Greek philosopher Socrates, teacher of Plato and the key figure in most of his work, taught mostly by asking questions. Answering a series of questions often led his listeners through a train of thought that led to conclusions quite different from what they originally believed to be true. Consequently, teaching by asking questions that stimulate students to think and work things out for themselves from their previous experience and by logical deduction is known as the Socratic method or Socratic questioning. In contrast to didactic teaching (lecturing) it ensures that the learner is actively engaged in the process. Note that Socratic questioning helps students to expand their understanding or work out the implications of what they already know; it should not be confused with an interrogation or a *viva voce* examination in which questions are asked to test the extent of a student's factual knowledge.

To read more visit: www.umich.edu/~elements/probsolv/strategy/cthinking.htm.

Virtue ethics

Virtue ethics puts moral character rather than rules (deontology) or maximising the good (consequentialism) at the centre of deciding how to live. Virtue ethicists argue that the cultivation of the virtues, the habit of acting rightly according to reason, is not only the best way to decide what one should do but is also the route to flourishing (*eudaemonia*): the best life to live.

Virtue was a central strand in ethical thinking in Ancient Greece and throughout the Middle Ages, but following the Enlightenment it received less attention from philosophers. There has been a renaissance in virtue ethics in the late twentieth century, much of which draws on the ideas of Aristotle. Prominent philosophers writing on virtue in recent decades include Philippa Foot, Rosalind Hursthouse, Martha Nussbaum, James Opie Urmson and of course Alasdair MacIntyre on whose seminal book *After Virtue* this work is based.

To read more visit: http://plato.stanford.edu/entries/ethics-virtue.

Index

Lightning Source UK Ltd.
Milton Keynes UK
UKOW05f1056150915

258669UK00001B/11/P